Fit for Riding

Fit for Riding

Exercises for Riders and Vaulters

Eckart Meyners
Translated by Elke Herrmann

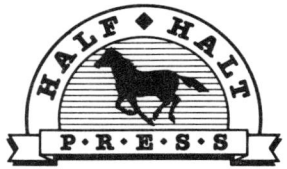

Half Halt Press, Inc.
Middletown, Maryland

Fit for Riding

Published by Half Halt Press, Inc.,
6416 Burkittsville Road, Middletown, MD 21769.

First published in Germany as **Fit aufs Pferd: Gymnastik fur Reiter und Voltigierer.**

© 1986 Jahr-Verlag GmbH & Co., Hamburg

This English transation

© 1992 Half Halt Press, Inc.

All rights reserved. No part of this book may be reproduced in any way or by any means without permission in writing from the Publisher.

Cover photo by Jacques Toffi

Translated by Elke Herrmann

Library of Congress Cataloging-in-Publication Data

Meyners, Eckart.
  [Fit aufs Pfers. English]
  Fit for riding / Eckart Meyners : translated by Elke Herrmann.
     p.   cm.
  ISBN 0-939481-29-4 : $18.95
  1. Horsemanship—Training. 2. Vaulting (Horsemanship)—Training.
3. Exercise. I. Title.
SF309.M5513 1992
798.2'4—dc20   92-34931
                                                                     CIP

Contents

Theoretical Part

I. Training and Conditioning 9
1.1   What is training 9
1.2   What is conditioning? 9
1.2.1 Speed 9
1.2.2 Strength 10
1.2.3 Endurance 10
1.2.4 Flexibility 11
1.2.5 Coordination 11

II What Basic Conditioning Do Riders and Vaulters Need? 12
2.1   Conditioning for riders 12
2.2   Conditioning for vaulters 13
2.3   Number and frequency of repitions 13

III General Training Principles 14
3.1   Correlation of form and function in the body 14
3.2   Finding the right amount of exercise for you 14
3.3   Capacity and training schedule 15
3.4   Amount of training 15
3.5   Stepping up your program 15
3.6   How often should I train? 16
3.7   Building up your program 16
3.8   A long-term training plan 16
3.9   Never mind what your friend does—
      you need your own program 16
3.10 Age 17
3.11 Special conditioning 17

IV Training Methods 17
4.1   Starting out 17
4.2   The circuit method 18
4.2.1 Establishing the right circuit for you 19
4.2.2 A general program (for working with a group) 19

V. Warm Up 20
5.1 Circulation 20
5.2 Body temperature 21
5.3 Warming up and breathing 21
5.4 Warming up to avoid injury 21
5.5 Improving coordination 21
5.6 Improving psychological performance 21

VI Different Kinds of Warm Ups 23
6.1 General warm up 22
6.2 Specific warm ups 22
6.3 Mental warm ups 23
6.4 Passive warm ups 23

VII Age—Again 23

VIII Practical Tips for Teaching Riding and Vaulting 25

Practical Part

Part I: General Conditioning
Strengthening exercises #1-28 30
Stretching exercises #29-40 59
Flexibility exercises #41-50 75
Coordination exercises #51-59 85

Part II: Additional exercises for riders
Strengthening exercises #60-72 95
Stretching exercises #73-81 109
Flexibility and coordination exercises #82-90 119

Part III: Additional exercises for vaulting
Strengthening exercises #91-100 129
Stretching exercises #101-106 141
Flexibility and coordination exercises #107-120 149

Foreword

In vaulting, the focus of the training is on the rider. In riding on the flat or over fences, however, most people see the horse as the one who must be trained and fit. But only a fit rider can give maximum support to the horse and guide it to high performance levels. This book is designed to help vaulters and riders improve their fitness properly and systematically by training the groups of muscles needed in their sports. A theoretical section about general aspects of training is followed by practical exercises.

Part I deals with general conditioning, which is important for both riders and vaulters. Part II contains special exercises for the rider, Part III for the vaulter. All of the exercises can be practiced during riding lessons as well as while schooling at home. The rider or coach may choose exercises, tailoring the exercise program for specific fitness goals. The exercises can be practiced easily and without special equipment. You should vary your program to combat boredom, just as you do your horse's. A varied program also is important for exercising different muscle groups and for working on physical fitness from different angles.

The goal is to get riders and vaulters interested in preparing better for the sport, just as athletes in other disciplines do. If you are prepared, success will come faster and more easily, and your horse will benefit.

1. Training and Conditioning

1.1 What Is Training?

We practice and exercise to improve riding or vaulting skills. We train to improve fitness or conditioning for riding or vaulting so that we can repeat the same exercise or movement several times without tiring. Repetitive training is useful for one lesson, one competition, or an entire season.

Training gives us *speed, strength,* and *endurance,* increases our physical performances in those areas, and helps us attain such qualities as *elasticity* and *speed and strength endurance.* Training also increases our *mechanical extension, flexibility,* and *coordination.* It helps to work with a coach at the beginning, but it is not a necessity. It is not difficult to determine the kind and extent of training yourself: Follow a regular routine, discipline yourself to build up gradually and systematically, and set goals. Remember, riders should use the exercises for riders, and vaulters the exercises for vaulters. Your age also will play an important role in determining your warm-up program.

1.2 What Is Conditioning?

Conditioning refers to the body's ability to be productive. This book looks at the physical aspects of conditioning (Figure 1); the psychological aspects go beyond the framework of this book.

It is important to make a distinction between general and special conditioning. The goal of general conditioning is even development of the entire body, whereas special conditioning focuses on getting fit for a particular sport. At the beginning of each workout, you should aim for all-around physical training and concentrate later on the special aspects of riding or vaulting. This principle is good for all training: Start with general exercises and then move to the special ones.

1.2.1 Speed

Speed refers to the ability to execute moves at short intervals and it depends on the interaction of the brain and the muscles. If certain moves cannot be made fast enough, the brain lacks flexibility. If the demand (stress) is very high (like holding a partner while vaulting, or riding a powerful, stubborn horse), you'll depend on your strength for speed in making the moves. That's what's known as *speed of action.*

Speed of reaction means the rider or vaulter reacts quickly to stimuli to eyes, ears, skin, sense of balance, or muscles. In riding and vaulting, you have to make certain moves over and over again over a long period of time. What you need is called *speed endurance.* Speed endurance allows you to repeat the same movements and to repeat them properly each time. Your body has to be able to replenish its muscles with oxygen while repeating the same moves quickly. When your oxygen is limited, your muscles get sore. Your arms and legs will feel heavy, they won't be as flexible, and some of the moves you make will be weak and faulty. Muscle soreness can be overcome with special methods of exercising.

1.2.2 Strength

Strength is the ability of the muscles to contract or to overcome resistance (that powerful, stubborn horse). We'll be talking about three kinds of strength: *maximum strength, elasticity* (elastic strength), and *enduring strength.*

Maximum strength is the greatest strength that you have. Elasticity refers to the ability of your brain to work with the muscles to allow you to move quickly—to get on the horse in vaulting, "scissors," to close your knees in critical jumping situations, or to increase your weight and leg aids when jumping combinations. Strength endurance calls for speed endurance, but also allows your body to withstand overtiredness during long periods of exercise and training.

1.2.3 Endurance

When your body has enough oxygen to make the moves you want to make, you have *aerobic endurance,* a balance of oxygen intake and expenditure of energy. People reach this balance when the pulse rate is under 140 beats per minute. Riders and vaulters need a high degree of aerobic endurance. The greater your aerobic endurance, the better you can develop your speed and strength endurance.

You rely on your aerobic endurance to execute properly the movements that require speed and strength endurance. When you execute movements calling for great strength and speed, you are working at 80 percent of maximum performance level. You'll be taking in little or no oxygen, expending energy you cannot replenish, so you will suffer from an oxygen deficiency. The longer you can do that, the more you develop aerobic endurance. When your pulse hits 180 beats per minute or more, you'll have hit your performance limit.

Open-jumper riders take a course in about a minute and come back puffing and sweating. They push over the fences and hold their breath (and so do the horses). They use a lot of oxygen that cannot be replenished while on course. To be successful, they have to condition their bodies to tolerate periods of great oxygen demand without suffering drops in performance. Difficult partner exercises in vaulting make similar demands on the body.

Special endurance is the ability to reach a high performance level quickly and it's different for each of the equestrian disciplines. A dressage rider needs special endurance or strength in the legs to ensure the "breathing leg." The jumper or event rider needs strength to maintain a light seat.

1.2.4 Flexibility

Agility is often described as joint mobility, suppleness, and flexibility. Essentially, agility means flexibility—the ability of a joint to have the greatest freedom of movement that the physiology of the joint allows.

In a broader sense, agility means to be nimble, an element of which is the monitoring of the muscles' movements by the brain. A rider or vaulter is agile when all joints are working freely and moving with ease. Agility can be limited by the structure of your body: the way your joints are built, the arrangement of your tendons and ligaments, the length, elasticity, and expandability of your muscles, and particularly if you are overweight. Agility is also influenced by your age, your outlook, your degree of fatigue, the outside temperature, time of day, or your method of warming up.

1.2.5 Coordination

Coordination is the interplay of muscles. Riders and vaulters must be highly coordinated—they need coordination to learn, to steer, and to be adaptable and flexible.

Coordination allows you to learn a movement quickly, to store the information, and to execute what you've learned in a given situation. In reacting to a situation you are coordinating your eyes, your ears, and your skin, and you are transmitting a sense of balance to your muscles. Coordination for steering includes your senses of orientation, balance and the resulting use of special muscles. If you are adaptable and flexible, you can make the right moves under various conditions and in changing situations.

You'll be working on five other coordination skills as well: orientation to space, sense of balance, reaction time, sense of rhythm, and muscular coordination. Orientation to space means that you can see your body in relation to the environment and time, and you can judge your moves for distance and obstacles. As you know, you need to be able to maintain your sense of balance, even when your center of gravity changes—when a horse knocks down a jump or a vaulting horse takes a wrong step. If you have good reaction time, it means you can react to a certain event quickly and with an appropriate move. This is the ability you call on to react to a signal or when something unexpected happens—your horse slips or your partner makes a mistake during a group vaulting exercise. Your sense of rhythm comes into play with a change from relaxed to tense movements: Posting to the trot or standing on a horse. Muscular coordination allows you to impart a high degree of accuracy and finesse to your movements.

2. What Basic Conditioning Do Riders and Vaulters Need?

2.1 Conditioning for Riders

A rider needs general aerobic endurance. All of your skills and abilities depend on it. The more oxygen you take in, the longer you can ride without tiring. General conditioning exercises train the rider's body as extensively as possible. These exercises can be done in circuits to achieve aerobic endurance (See Exercises, Part I). Jogging works, too, but you'll have to do it for at least 20 minutes to reach a pulse of 140 to 150, which encourages your cardiovascular system to adjust to an even higher energy demand. Increase the time and distance after three or four weeks to increase your strength and endurance.

When you've reached the point that you've achieved good, basic conditioning, you can add the special riding exercises. Dressage, jumping, and eventing require special aids that have to be applied over long periods of time without tiring. They have to be given to the horse quickly, and they must be firm and continuous. You need speed and strength endurance to apply the aids with your leg, back, stomach and arm muscles. You need to be agile so you can move with your horse.

Since the rider needs a fine-tuned interplay of all the muscles, you have to exercise for it constantly. You have to be able to coordinate your back, legs, and arms to give aids smoothly and quietly; this kind of coordination is particularly difficult because you often will be using cross movements— right leg, left shoulder.

2.2 Conditioning for Vaulters

The vaulter, too, needs good, general conditioning. In addition, the compulsory and kur exercises demand speed, strength, mobility, elasticity, and coordination (especially for partner exercises). Basic conditioning for vaulting cannot be accomplished by exercising only on the vaulting horse; you need to supplement your program with floor exercises, which can be done in the gym or on a horse blanket in the arena. Vaulters need extra mobility and elasticity, for example, for the "scissors" or the "mill," which must be done in large, swinging circles. Many exercises (basic seat, mill, scissors) require you to spread and stretch your arms and legs, while others (standing on the horse and "flag") require balance. The more you have exercised for these abilities on the floor, the better you'll be able to do them on the horse.

2.3 Number and Frequency of Repetitions

Believe it or not, body-building is comparable to riding and vaulting. All require a certain number of repetitions in order to reach the conditioning goal. For speed and elasticity, exercises should be repeated up to 10 times. For speed and endurance, repeat them 20 to 30 times. To achieve general aerobic conditioning, exercises like jumping rope should be done 40 to 60 or more times.

We all start out in different conditions, so it's impossible to prescribe a certain number of exercises. What's too much for one person is too little for another. You might want to start by working with a trainer at a gym who can give you a conditioning test. But if you are working on your own, the rule is this: Once you've figured out how to do each exercise in the front of the book, repeat them frequently. Those are the exercises for general, aerobic endurance and that's what riders and vaulters must achieve first.

To add agility and coordination to speed and strength endurance, repeat the special exercises at least 15 times each. Your performance level and coordination will increase only if you've done the maximum number of repetitions frequently and regularly.

These exercises require hard work—they guarantee a good supply of blood to the muscles. Riders and vaulters mainly need these "dynamic" or isotonic exercises; isometric or static exercises are secondary. The isometric, or strength, exercises narrow the blood vessels and therefore slow the blood supply. They also require pressing and tensing, which have some negative effects that will be dealt with later.

3. General Training Principles

There are certain training principles—laws, rules, and methods—that have to be followed in the daily routine to ensure success.

3.1 Correlation of Form and Function in the Body

The structures of organs and their functions are mutually dependent. For example, heart volume is directly related to endurance. Certain exercises can increase the volume and strengthen the heart muscle, allowing the rider or vaulter to overcome tiredness during long stretches of riding, schooling, or competition.

3.2 Finding the Right Amount of Exercise for You

You can exercise every day, but that does not mean you're getting the right results. What you are seeking is a program that works you at 80 percent of the maximum that your current physical condition will allow you to do.

If you exercise too much—if you do 90 percent or more of what you can possibly do in your current condition—you're not going to feel very well, and you may do yourself some harm. You'll feel sore and tired, your coordination will be shot, and you'll be all too aware that if something unexpected happens, you won't be able to rely on your body to react properly.

On the other hand, if you exercise too little—if you do, say, 30 percent of what you could possibly do—you won't be achieving anything. You won't even be able to prevent decay of the condition of your current.

Of course, what you will be able to do as a result of an exercise program depends on what your training goal is. When you are ready to step up your program, you want to do it at 80 percent of your capacity. For endurance training, you should be working at 50 to 60 percent of capacity.

But how do you calculate your capacity?

If you can do an exercise only 10 times in a row, you have to repeat it during training at least 8 times to train the specific muscle groups and you have to do it often (repetitions). If your best time for running 100 meters is 12 seconds, you have to be able to maintain a speed of 24 seconds per 100 meters (50 percent of maximum speed) for 20 minutes to achieve endurance.

3.3 Capacity and Training Schedule

As you ride or vault, your energy level drops. The loss of energy requires a recovery period. It is important to maintain the right balance between work-out and recovery. If you maintain a proper training schedule over a long period of time, you will achieve greater efficiency (Figure 2). If you increase your training slowly, you'll get maximum benefit from each session and increase your performance (Figure 3). But your performance will deteriorate if you exercise too much and don't rest enough afterward (Figure 4).

3.4 Amount of Training

As your performance improves, your progress will slow down. At first, a little bit of exercise will create noticeable improvements in your performance and in how you feel. And the greater your training goal is, the more you have to train just to maintain the conditioning you have achieved. Later in the training process, you'll be working hard, but seeing only a little bit of improvement (Figure 5).

3.5 Stepping Up Your Program

At first, exercise causes a lot of stress reactions that become less noticeable, even barely noticeable, as your conditioning improves. It follows, therefore, that you can improve your performance only by incremental increases in how much you are exercising. Because your body adjusts to the stress of training, you have to check from time to time on how much training you are doing. For example, if you jog twice a week for one hour, after three or four weeks, you'll have to jog farther and longer or increase the frequency to experience the original amount of stress. Paradoxically, increasing your exercise time means that you need less rest between workouts—the more fit you become, the faster your body recovers.

3.6 How Often Should I Train?

Training once a week does not increase performance; at best, it maintains your training level. Training every two weeks won't do anything for you. And if you train less than that, you won't even have the strength to overcompensate.

Your goal should be to train several times a week and the frequency should be increased systematically over several years.

3.7 Building Up Your Program

Training goals cannot be attained overnight; they need to be built up over years. If a rider or vaulter trains gradually, the drop in performance level is much slower if, for example, an injury requires rest. A quick build-up always leads to a quick decline of performance if training stops. A slow build-up is far more enduring.

3.8 A Long-term Training Plan

Some training methods are monotonous and you'll be bored. Some repetitive exercises (the ones you already know) are hard to give up. But monotony is the worst thing to tolerate because it decreases your ability to adapt to new techniques and to be flexible in dealing with new situations. Therefore, it's important to constantly strive for a changing program.

3.9 Never Mind What Your Friend Does— You Need Your Own Program

Everyone is different, so we need different programs to address different problems and abilities. You need to pay attention to your strong points as well as your weak ones. If you have good aerobic endurance, you can concentrate on other needs—but don't lose sight of aerobic endurance. Also, we each have different priorities and goals. A dressage rider needs agility and coordination in addition to good basic conditioning. An event rider needs extra endurance—general endurance and speed and strength endurance—especially for the cross-country day. If these basics of conditioning for event riding are neglected, the rider does not have total body control and the horse is burdened with the rider's weight in addition to the demands of the course.

3.10 Age
A child or a teenager needs different conditioning (general endurance, for one) than does a twenty-year-old dressage rider. The same is true for vaulters.

3.11 Special Conditioning
Performance-oriented conditioning for riding and vaulting is divided into three phases—basic, intermediate, and advanced—and follows a training plan of several (four or five or more) years. The basic training program for children and teenagers covers a systematic build-up for general fitness. The basics should be acquired slowly and steadily increased in order to have a solid base to build on later. This is followed by conditioning that involves the intense development of special abilities, depending on the discipline—dressage, jumping, eventing, or vaulting.

Advanced (high performance) training means to train for performance at the highest demand. Rider and horse have to be physically and mentally at the peak of fitness. And the rider has to have a fire in the belly, without which success can not be attained.

4. Training Methods

4.1 Starting Out
This method is marked by relatively low intensity—you'll be working at about 50 percent of your capacity. That means you'll have to jog for 24 seconds per 100 meters to reach a maximum speed of 12 seconds per 100 meters. Average jogging speed is individual. Because of the relatively low demand, you can maintain an average speed over longer distances to increase your capacity. If the distance is great, your body will be highly stimulated. You might need to walk for brief periods. If you jog more slowly than your average speed, but go farther, you can stretch your program from a half hour to one hour. Your pulse will tell you if you have

reached aerobic endurance—it should not be less than 140 or 150.

If for some reason you cannot jog, you can do the exercises in the first part of this book for a longer period of time without resting. Do the exercises consecutively, so you don't stress the same group of muscles all the time, which might lead to over-training. To achieve aerobic endurance, you might want to use the circuit method (see below). You'll know you're adapting to the program when you find your pulse is returning to normal faster than it did after you first began the exercise program. Another proof of improved performance is if your resting pulse rate is lower than it was before you started a training program. A lowered pulse rate means that your heart is carrying more volume now that you are in condition; before, your heart had to beat more often to produce the same result.

4.2 The Circuit Method

The main characteristics of the circuit method are:
—Improvement of muscle strength and circulation
—Greater capacity for exercise
—Accommodation of many athletes at the same time

This training method is similar to the body-building system in which the athlete rotates from station to station to do exercises. The order of exercises in a circuit need not follow a circle, but there should be no consecutive exercises that work the same muscles.

The content of the circuit training program depends on the goal (aerobic endurance or enduring strength, for example). The amount of training depends on the individual and must be readjusted continually to allow for progress. Short, intensive circuits with long rest periods, for example, do not result in aerobic endurance. Aerobic endurance is the result of sustained exercises for the heart. Because circuit training calls for exercises to be done in quick succession, an athlete will not reach maximum capacity with any single exercise. But you can reach your training goal through the cumulative effect of the exercises. A single circuit is not very demanding, but several circuits can be.

In designing a circuit, you have to know the purpose of each exercise. The exercises should be arranged so that your body is under constantly changing stress, doing different arm and shoulder exercises, working the abdominal muscles, working different leg muscles, and working the body as a whole.

The ingredients of the circuit depend on the goal. An easy circuit leads to aerobic endurance, a difficult one to strength and speed endurance.

Each circuit should last at least 10 minutes (a short circuit) and no more than 30 minutes (a long circuit).

Furthermore, the demand of the circuit should not be so great that you are exhausted, for example, after three rounds and must have a long rest period. Use specific and general amounts of exercise in increments to get the right combination.

4.2.1 Establishing the Right Circuit for You

There are three steps in establishing the right circuit and right number of circuits for you: Learn the exercises, figure out what your maximum capacity for each exercise is at the moment, and time how long it takes you to complete one circuit.

You need to understand what each exercise does for you (which muscles it works), how to do it and how to do it correctly. You should be able to do each circuit one to three times without becoming totally exhausted. And have fun with it. (If you are working with a group of people, this process can take an hour or more.)

After two or three training sessions, test yourself on the number of times you can comfortably repeat each exercise in the circuit. Then cut the number of repetitions of each exercise in half to give you your base training level for the circuit. The time that it took you to complete three circuits is the time that you should spend during each exercise session.

After some time—and that time is specific to you—you will find that you are finishing each circuit faster than you once did. That's the cumulative effect of training—it's working! Now it's time to test yourself again, again cutting in half the number of repetitions you can comfortably do and limiting the number of circuits to three.

The other way to approach it is to leave the number of repetitions and circuits the same as in your starting program, but to start pushing yourself to complete each circuit faster.

4.2.2 A General Program (for working with a group)

This method of basic training is easier, but requires that you work in a group that has roughly common training goals and roughly equal levels of fitness. With this method, it is important to do the three circuits quickly. You need to establish how long you will be at each station and the length of your breaks. The goal is to increase the number of times you repeat each exercise and; therefore, the overall number of exercises you will do. The number of exercises and the lengths of your breaks depend on your goal. For example, for aerobic endurance, you want to do the first exercise for 30 seconds, the second for 45 seconds and the third for 60 seconds. Then you get a 30-second break. For strength endurance, take a 45- to 60-second break (or more) after each 30 seconds of exercise. (The break period gets longer if your need for oxygen increases, as in efforts that require speed or strength endurance.) The exercise and break periods have to be planned according to your pulse (for aerobic endurance, you want to hit 140 to 150 beats per minute; for anaerobic endurance, 180 beats per minute or more). You (or your trainer) have to take your pulse constantly so you know how you are doing.

Which ever method you choose, remember that your increased fitness is demonstrated by your ability to do more work in the same period of time, or by doing a certain amount of work faster than you once did. Remember, too, that you'll see a lot of improvement at first, and then your improvement will slow down.

5. Warm up

Not warming up is something most riders are guilty of, although vaulters are becoming more aware of the need to warm up. There probably are very few riders who warm up before tests or lessons or who go to the gym regularly, in addition to riding, to improve strength, speed, endurance, agility, and coordination.

Although there have been specific warm-up programs for years in track and field, soccer, football, and other sports, riders have not yet realized how important it is for them to stretch and warm their muscles before they mount.

5.1 Circulation

Warming up increases the amount of blood that supplies the muscles with the oxygen and nourishment needed for riding. Metabolic waste, which burdens muscles, is taken away, preventing muscle soreness. That allows the rider or vaulter to work for longer periods.

It also is important for the intensive blood supply of the capillary system, the fine vessels right under the skin, to get a better oxygen supply.

5.2 Body Temperature

Warming up makes your body's temperature (which should be 98.6 degrees Fahrenheit) rise. Because the temperature in your arms, hands, legs, and feet can be lower than 98.6 (especially on cold days), it's easy to see how important warming up is for those body parts because we rely on them so much in riding and vaulting.

5.3 Warming Up and Breathing

The tempo and depth of your breathing increases during your warm-up to give your muscles more oxygen and to take the carbon dioxide away. Normally, your breathing increases just after the warm-up begins. As you continue to warm up, you'll soon reach a point where you are breathing rapidly but evenly. Warming up increases your breathing so that your regulating mechanisms are humming by the time you actually start to exercise.

5.4 Warming Up to Avoid Injury

When your body temperature rises, your muscles don't rub against each other (friction) and your risk of injury is reduced. Warming up also makes your muscles more elastic and your whole body becomes more mobile. Low outside temperatures can disturb your mobility and coordination, increasing the risk of injury if you don't warm up first.

5.5 Improving Coordination

With less friction and more elasticity, different muscles and muscle groups coordinate better. Improved coordination means you'll need less energy to do what you want to do and you won't get tired as fast. Warming up also relaxes you, which is good for your muscles. And with higher body temperature, your brain reflexes work faster.

5.6 Improving Psychological Performance

Warming up also reduces the anxiety of the rider or vaulter. It has a positive effect on the psyche. Older riders need to warm up more slowly and more deliberately than younger people do. We get less elastic as we get older, so our risk of injury is greater. And it takes longer to warm up in the morning than it does in the evening. But our overall performance decreases throughout the day. It takes longer to warm up in colder temperatures than it does in warm ones, and if it's cold, you need to dress more warmly. The more fit you get in your exercise program, the longer and harder your warm up should be—it increases the effect.

6. Different Kinds of Warm ups

Different kinds of warm-ups emphasize different aspects and produce different reactions from your body.

6.1 General Warm up

A general warm-up prepares large groups of muscles, not necessarily the ones you need for specific activities. It involves your whole body in order to increase your overall performance. The exercises have to be repeated often to get your cardiovascular system charged up and they have to be increased slowly to get the body to optimum temperature (101.3 to 102.2 degrees). To avoid overtaxation, do not exercise the same muscles or groups of muscles several times in a row. The exercises should work different parts of the body progressively, rather than the same ones frequently.

6.2 Specific Warm ups

To warm up specifically for riding and vaulting, we have to be sure that each exercise consists of stretching, loosening, and strengthening the muscles. The exercises should keep body temperature at 101.3 to 102.2 degrees.

Our muscles are often cramped and tense, so we should start with stretching to loosen the long muscles enough so that they can receive and transport impulses of the brain. Strengthening exercises can follow. Then, you have to relax the muscles again, to avoid tension and a drop in performance. Keep moving between exercises by jogging or skipping to maintain your increased body temperature. It is difficult to say how often an exercise should be repeated—20 times can be too much for one person and not enough for another. But the exercises chosen for warm up should be easily repeatable 15 to 20 times.

6.3 Mental Warm ups

Mental warm up has no effect on body temperature and metabolism, but it's still important. What it means is that you should picture an exercise in your mind before you actually do it—it makes the exercise easier to do.

6.4 Passive Warm ups

There are ways to raise your body temperature without exercising: Hot showers, massages, and liniments. The body temperature does not rise, but the muscles loosen and the capillary system gets stimulated so it takes in more oxygen.

Training can enlarge the capillary system by as much as 145 percent. When working, the capillary system can take in 240 times the amount of oxygen as when resting, so it's important for performance, too. Combined warm ups, general and specialized, seem to be the most effective.

7. Age—Again

If you haven't learned a movement or a sport before puberty, it's difficult, if not impossible, to learn it later. That means that children should start riding or vaulting early so they can develop and refine their skills from puberty to adulthood. A latecomer who becomes very good at riding or vaulting is relying on skills learned much earlier in life in other disciplines, such as gymnastics, surfing, or skiing. A generally well-trained athlete has a better chance of succeeding at a new sport as an adult. The less balance riders and vaulters have, the more important it is to also engage in a conditioning program—it will even out weaknesses and lessen difficulties on horseback later on (See 1.25, Coordination).

Furthermore, it is important to learn movements correctly the first time. Mistakes are difficult—if not impossible—to eliminate later. Lack of conditioning is often the reason for wrong movements.

Children (11 for girls, 12 or 13 for boys) primarily need good general conditioning and good basic riding instruction. The more extensively and directly their coordination is trained, the better they will cope with acquiring advanced skills on horeseback. But it also is important to remember that children younger than eight often are not very coordinated—they can't always use their hands, arms, legs, and feet correctly. Those abilities develop and hit their first peak at 10 and 11. In addition to general training, it is important to work on flexibility and elasticity from the ages of 10 to 14 because those abilities cannot be improved upon later in life. Later efforts can only maintain the mobility of ages 10 to 14. Prepubescent boys and girls have the same abilities; occasional differences owe to early development. At puberty, those conditions change.

Children should not attempt difficult partner exercises because their spines are not yet protected with strong muscle systems. Straining exercises also should be avoided: When you hold your breath, blood is jammed in the veins, so the heart could slow down, pumping insufficient blood to the brain for the movement. A child could faint. Further, when a child who has been straining continues to breathe, blood enters the heart under increased pressure, and its rather thin walls could be damaged. This also is true for youngsters at puberty. Otherwise, the liveliness and joyousness of children offer positive psychological momentum for learning.

Teenagers. Puberty often leads to a decrease in mobility. It's rare to see a teenager's performance increase; it's best to maintain the mobility acquired in childhood. The reason for the drop in mobility is the rapid growth, first in height and then in bulk, of the teen's long bones. These are the changes that often make teenagers seem clumsy, which can be very inhibiting. A coach must be very careful and understanding—and not take anything that they say too seriously. The goal here is to maintain the coordination these young people had at 10 or 11. The main advantage teenage boys have over girls is strength. A 10- or 11-year-old can barely gain strength through exercise (the hormone testosterone is the basis for the growth of muscles), but the increased hormonal activity during the teen years means boys get stronger. Teenage girls are more flexible and mobile than their male counterparts. Therefore, a coach cannot expect the same performances of teenage girls and boys. The rapid growth in height can mean spinal weaknesses, so the coach has to watch the teen's development of a build as well as the body position. This is an especially good time for general conditioning—particularly of the muscles of the back, abdomen, arms, and legs—as well as special conditioning. But care must be taken with strengthening exercises: Growth gaps close at the end of puberty, so the bones are weak.

The late teen years are the time for increasing performance without problems; they also are the time for attaining peak performance. The body conditioning is good and height and bulk are in proportion. Special and focused conditioning—with the goals of speed and endurance—also can heighten performance.

Adults. We lose our anaerobic conditioning from the mid-30s on, so the rider should be anaerobically trained by then. The more solid the conditioning a rider has by the mid-30s, the more gradual will be the rider's loss of endurance, strength, mobility, and elasticity. As we age, we need to be careful not to abruptly neglect exercise because lack of strength, speed, and endurance automatically lead to a loss of coordination. In other words, a rider rides well only so long as he or she maintains overall physical fitness.

Today, more adults who barely exercised before take up riding, so conditioning is especially important. The more agile and fit they become, the easier latecomers will find riding a horse.

8. Practical Tips for Teaching Riding and Vaulting

Warm ups and fitness training can be done in various places. The exercises here were designed to be simple and were chosen because they do not require special rooms or equipment. The indoor arena, the outdoor ring (and surroundings) or any rooms connected to the arena can be used without difficulty. Many people can work in a small place, especially with circuit training. You can use horse blankets as floor mats to protect against cold or dirt. Some of the exercises for vaulters (depending on the goal) can be practiced on the horse. Youngsters who are not on horses can use the time to do other exercises.

All riders know to start their daily schooling slowly, to help their horses warm up and loosen up. But they themselves are not suitably warmed up, elastic, and supple. Yes, they warm up as they ride, but it is too late and counter-productive. Riders would make it easier for their horses if they warmed up before they mounted.

Chances are that you'll ride better if you warm up first. My work with riders and coaches has impressed me time and again with how important and helpful proper preparation can be. One group did a warm up program and followed it with sitting exercises. The riders and observers of the session reached the same conclusion: The riders felt better and more supple from the start; the observers saw better seats and positions. The conclusion is that a long-term, regular fitness training program improves the rider's seat and aids. However, riders and vaulters cannot rely only on weekly riding, but must use fitness training to constantly improve physical conditioning. How many times have you heard a coach yelling, "Chest out!" "Shoulder blades together!"? The faulty seats and positions could derive from weaknesses in the riders' bodies, which could be corrected by exercising the right muscle groups.

That's why this book contains the special exercises, in addition to those for general conditioning of riders and vaulters. They can be helpful, for example, in solving a rider's poor back position. An upright seat requires balanced relaxation of the back, shoulder, chest, leg, and stomach muscles, i.e., the cooperation of those five muscle groups. A rider's crooked position could be caused by weak back muscles because the more powerful muscles of the chest and stomach do not allow the rider to sit straight. As hard as the rider tries, whenever anything untoward happens, he or she always ends up in the wrong position. But the special exercises to intensively train the back muscles can correct such mistakes of position. If a rider has a weak back, seat, and leg muscles, the rider cannot sit the horse with confidence and often ends up "sitting behind the movement" (leaning back with the upper body) to compensate. There are similar situations in vaulting.

The following examples show that the exercises here serve the special needs of equestrian sports. An open-jumper rider has to have a light but firm seat. The rider's inner and outer thigh muscles must be equally strong for the rhythmical riding a big course demands. One exercise that does that is the one in which one person lies down and another person tries to open or close—with the supine person resisting—his or her thighs. Similarly, the dressage rider's "following, breathing leg" requires fully developed inner and outer muscles of the entire leg. Because riding requires coordinated movements, including the coordination of muscles from opposite sides of the body, the exercises here are designed to meet those demands, too.

Summary of Important Points:
—Continue to breathe while doing exercises that call for you to hold the position, so no tenseness develops in your muscles.

—Riders and vaulters should include isometric phases for riding and vaulting because both disciplines demand them in reality (to "sit against" a resistant horse, or the holding phases during partner exercises on the horse).

—Don't forget to regularly increase the number of strengthening exercises you do. Your speed and endurance depend on how often the exercise can be repeated.

—Work in this order: Stretching, loosening, strengthening, stretching. *Note:* Only a stretched long muscle can be loose and avoid tension. Also, stretching exercises do have a strengthening effect. The muscle opposite the stretched one gets strengthened (stretching the stomach strengthens the back). The exercise number indicates the order of the exercises. Your trainer determines the number of repetitions according to your level of fitness and your goals.

—If you are working with a trainer, the trainer must learn to use the exercises systematically. The trainer needs to teach you the positions and the reasons for the various exercises. Then you'll be able to do them on your own.

Practical Part I

General Conditioning

Strengthening Exercises

General Conditioning

Exercise No. 1

Strengthening Stomach Muscles

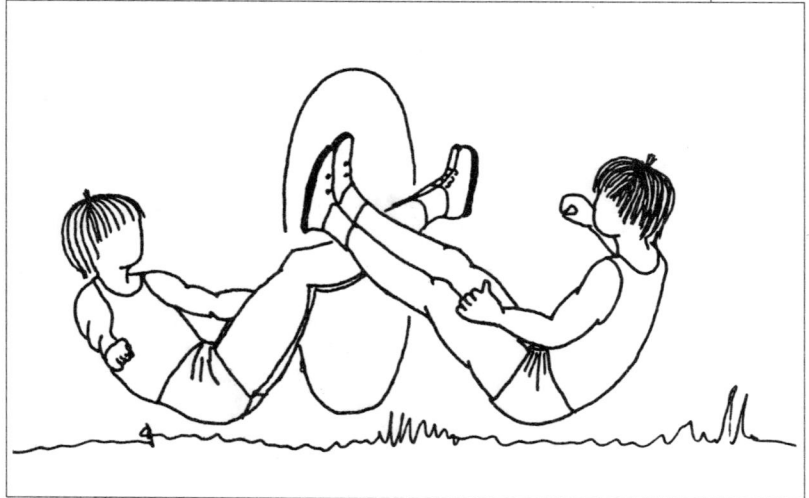

Leg circling: A circles her closed legs around the legs of B. **Note:** Make big circles, with arms in the air.

General Conditioning

Exercise No. 2

Strengthening Leg Muscles

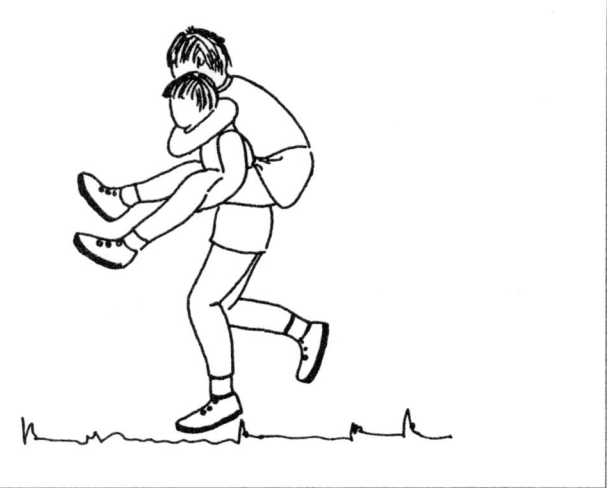

Trotting with a partner, piggy-back. **Note:** partners should have near equal weight!

General Conditioning

Exercise No. 3

Strengthening Stomach muscles
(front muscles)

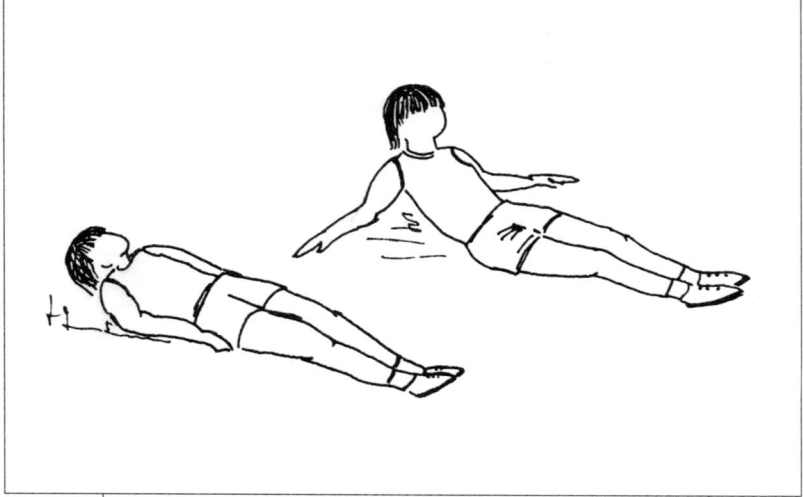

Lying on the back, lift the head while stretching the entire body to the tips of the toes.

General Conditioning

Exercise No. 4

Strengthening Stomach Muscles

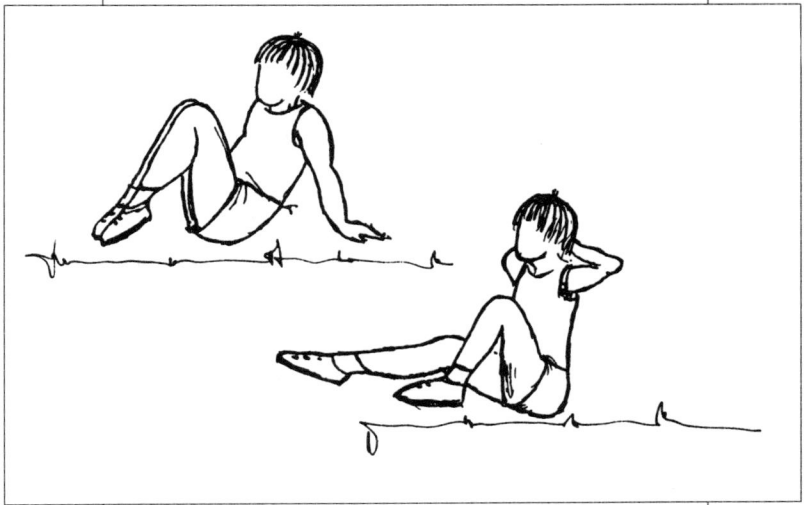

From a seated position, as shown, sit up; with hands behind head stretch on leg or both.

General Conditioning

Exercise No. 5

Strengthening Stomach Muscles

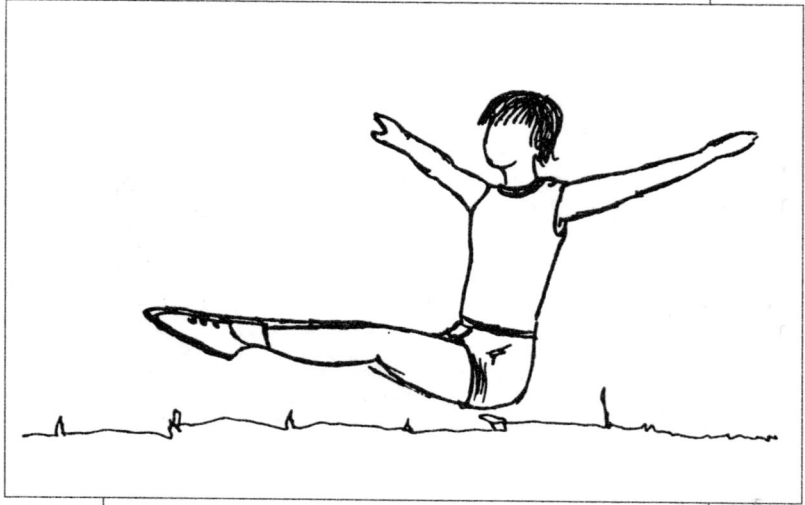

Balancing on buttocks and holding arms straight out, lift legs.

General Conditioning

Exercise No. 6

Strengthening
Stomach and Hip Muscles

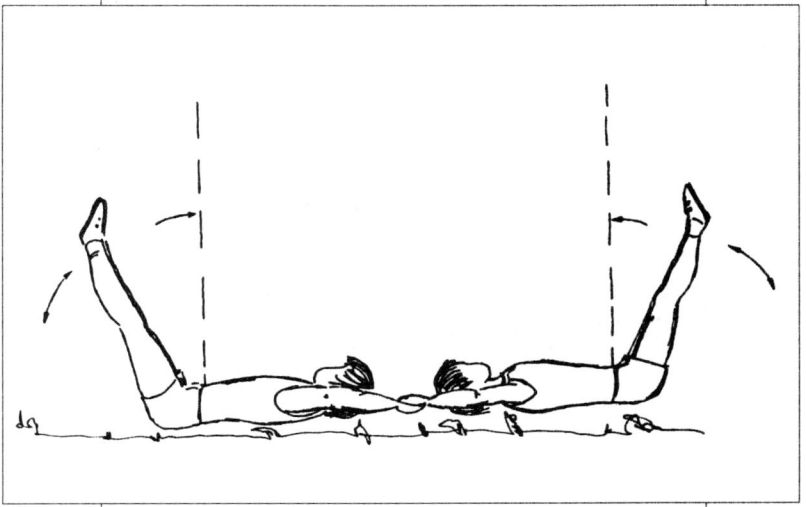

Both partners lie on their backs, head to head, arms on the floor, hands held: both lift up their legs to upright position and put them down slowly again.

General Conditioning

Exercise No. 7

Strengthening Stomach and Hip Muscles

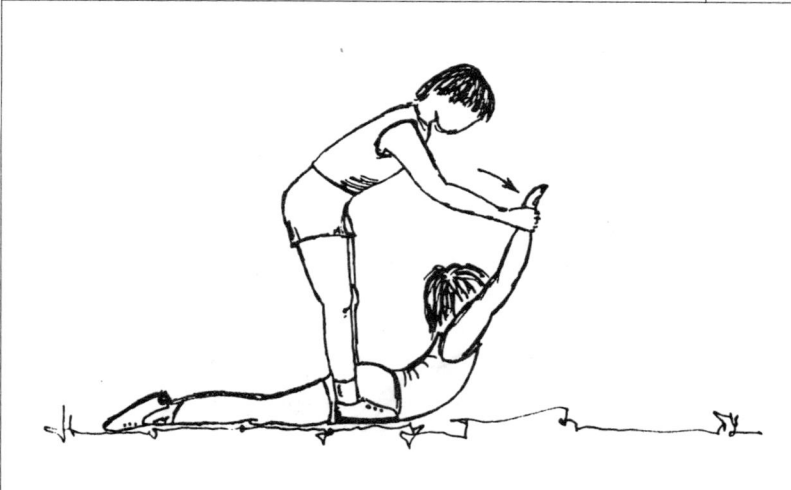

A lies on her tummy and lifts arms and upper torso. B offers resistance. She can apply the resistance on the arms or shoulder.

General Conditioning

Exercise No. 8

Strengthening
Back and Hip Muscles

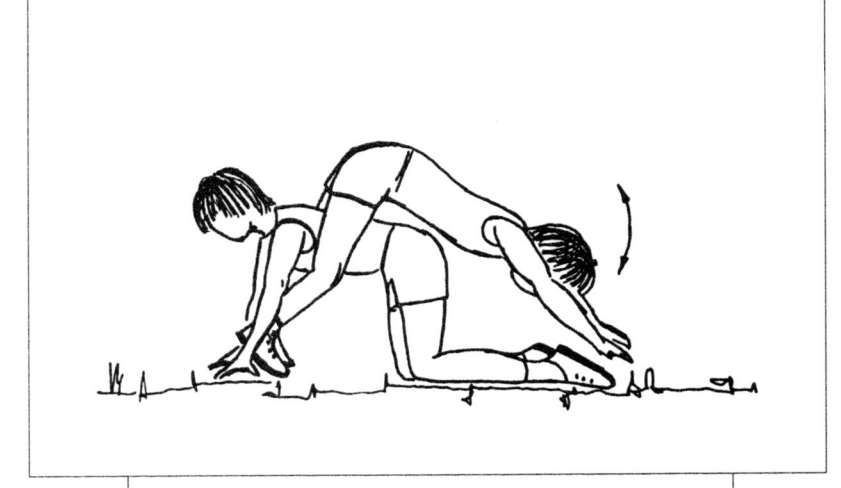

A is on her hands and knees, B lies on A's back and hooks her legs behind the arms of A, with her arms extended straight over her head. B then raises and lowers her upper torso.

General Conditioning

Exercise No. 9

Strengthening
Hip, Leg, and Stomach Muscles

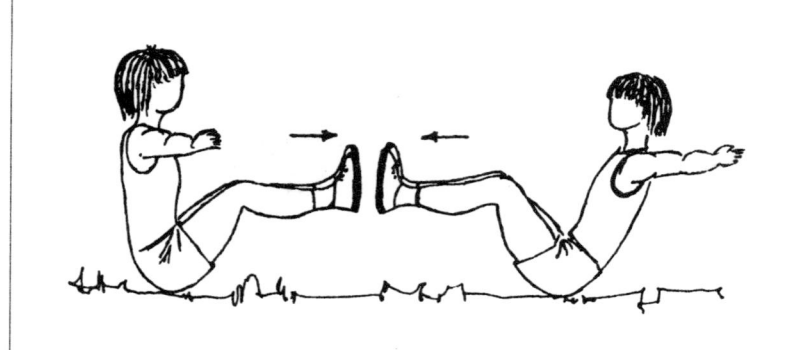

Partners sit opposite one another balanced on buttocks with bent legs and arms held sideways. They try to push each other over, pushing with their feet. By moving their feet right or left, they try to avoid the efforts of the other partner.

General Conditioning

Exercise No. 10

Strengthening
Back, Hip, and Shoulder Muscles

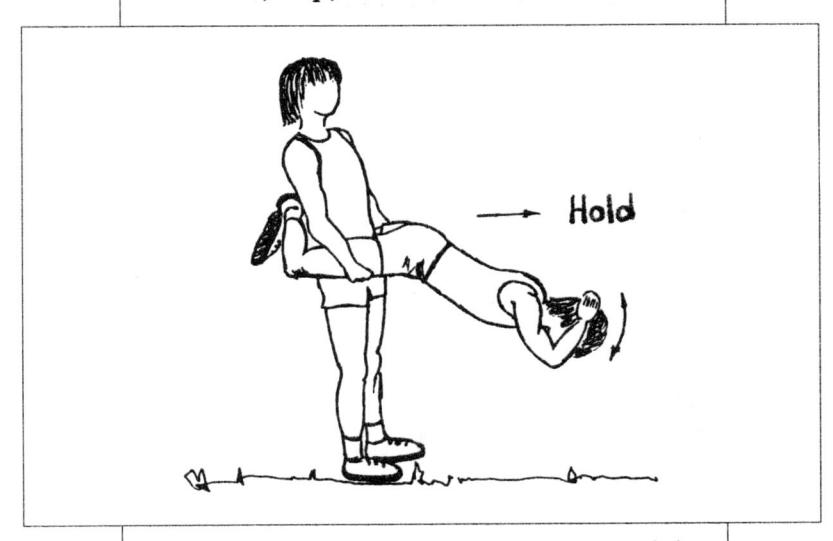

Hold

A crosses her legs behind the back of B who stands in straddling position behind her, and holds A on her thighs. A lifts and lowers her upper body, hands held on the neck.

General Conditioning

Exercise No. 11

Endurance for Leg Muscles, and General Endurance

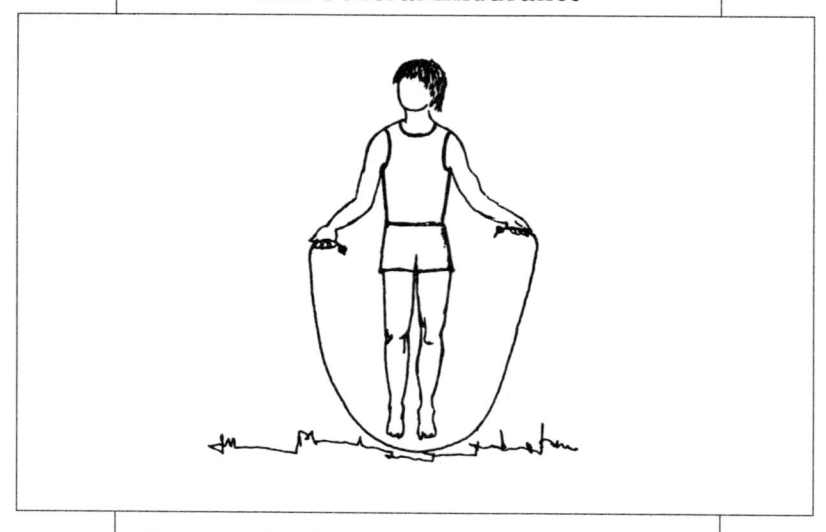

Jump rope: jumping with feet together.

General Conditioning

Exercise No. 12

Endurance for Leg Muscles, and General Endurance

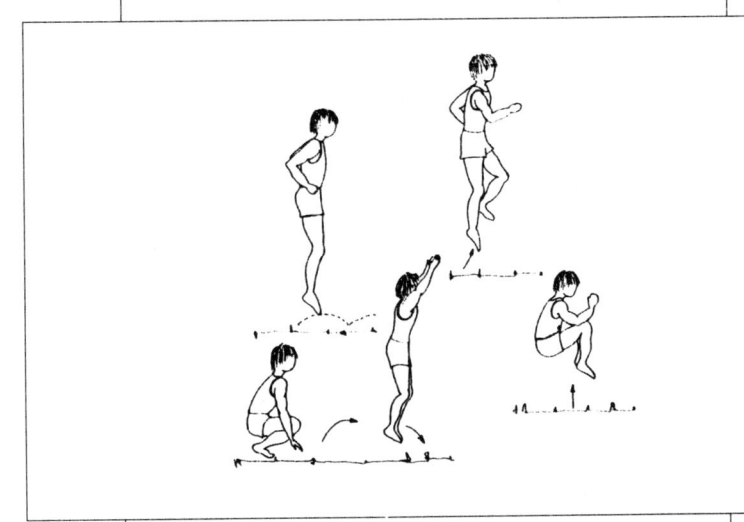

Jump forward, then do one-legged skipping, changing left/right leg forward, then do stretch jumps out of squatting position to stretched position, followed by jumping forward while squatting with both legs.

General Conditioning

Exercise No. 13

Strengthening the Body Muscles

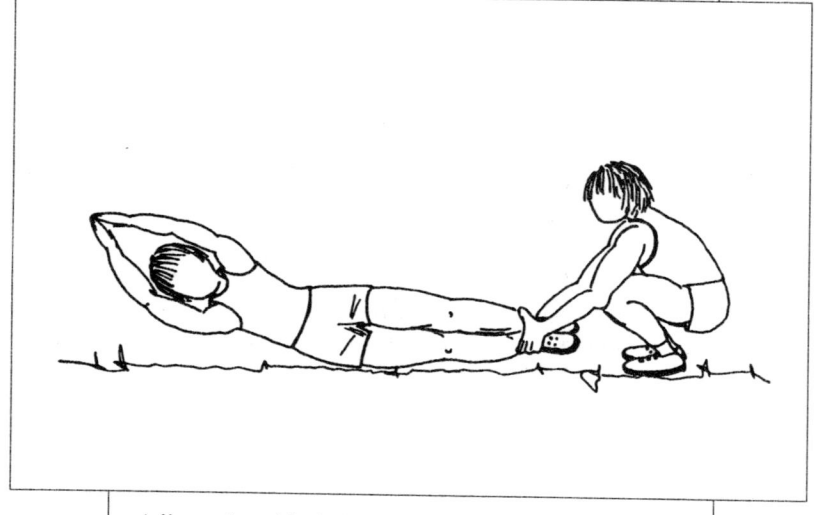

A lies on her side, holding her arms. B pushes the ankles of A onto the floor, as A lifts and lowers her upper body.

General Conditioning

Exercise No. 14

Strengthening Leg Muscles, Improving Coordination

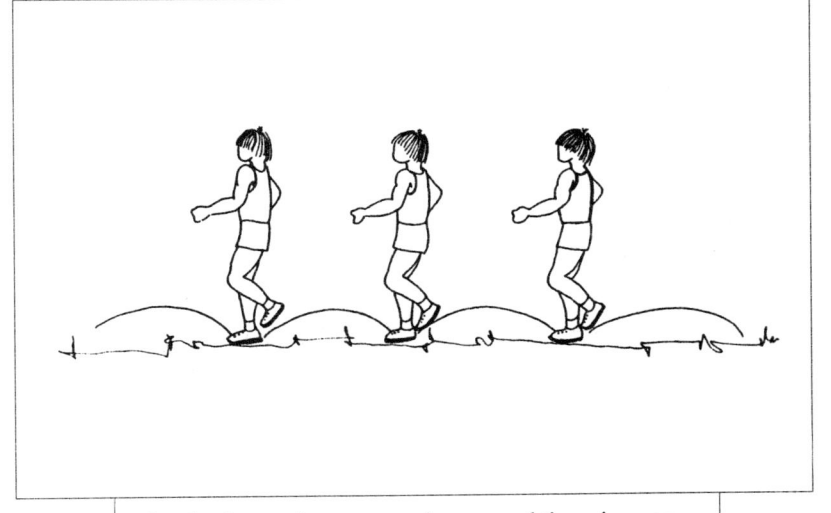

One leg jumps: jump on one leg, several times in a row, change leg. As ground is gained, pull up the thigh of the bent leg to a horizontal position.

General Conditioning

Exercise No. 15

Strengthening Back and Shoulder Muscles

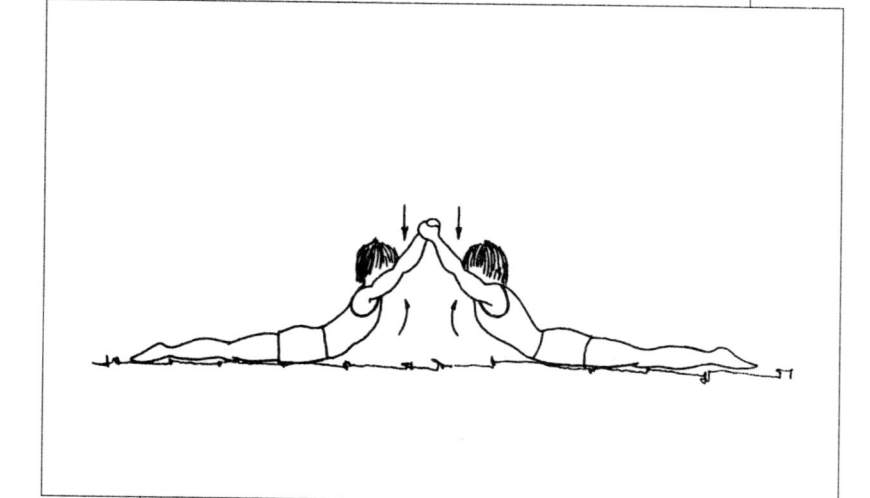

Both partners lie on their tummies facing each other, hands held and arms bent. They stretch arms at the same time propping each other up, then go back to starting position.

General Conditioning

Exercise No. 16

Strengthening Leg Muscles, Improving Coordination

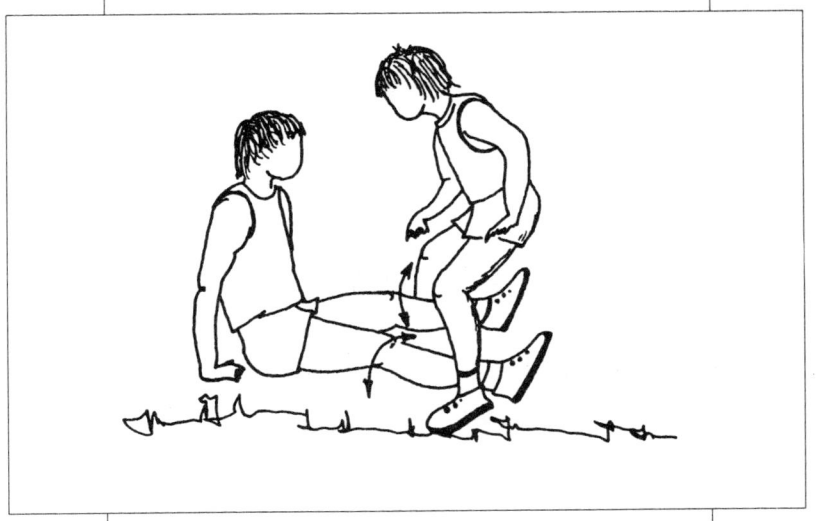

The straddling jump: outside to inside and vice versa.

General Conditioning

Exercise No. 17

Stretching and Strengthening Front Thigh Muscles and Stomach Muscles

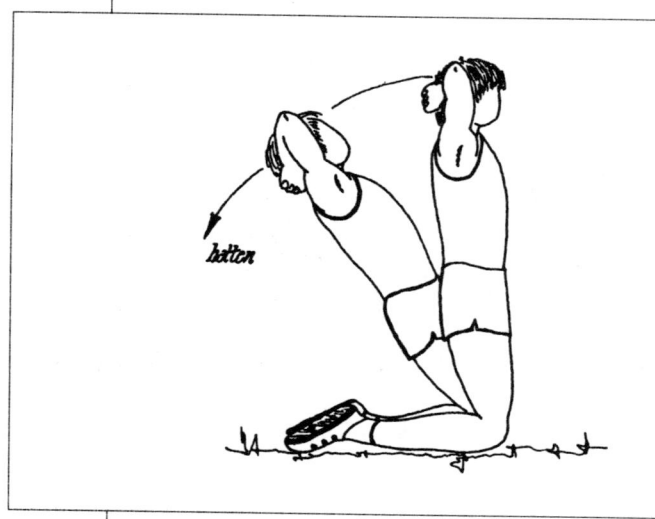

With upper body upright, bend body way back, holding for a moment, then straighten. Repeat exercise several times, *do not* sit down on your heels.

General Conditioning

Exercise No. 18

Strengthening Back Muscles, Improving Coordination

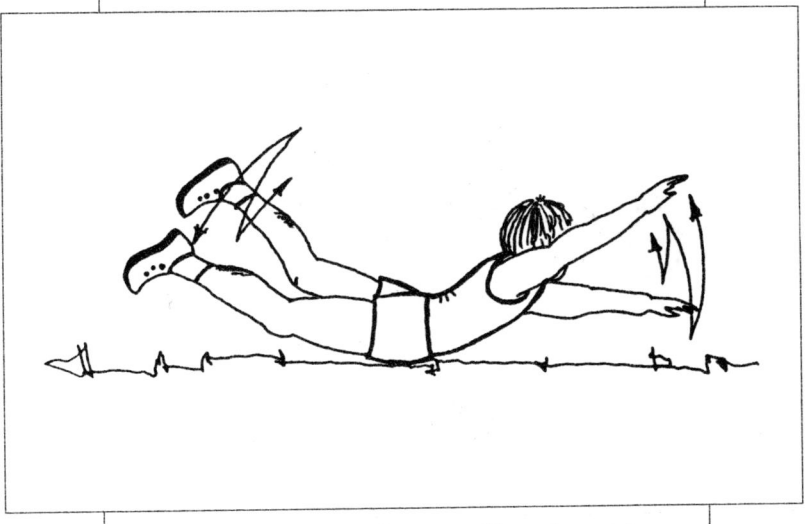

In the tummy position, lift arms and legs alternately up and down. The tempo can be varied.

General Conditioning

Exercise No. 19

Strengthening Upper Arm and Shoulder Muscles

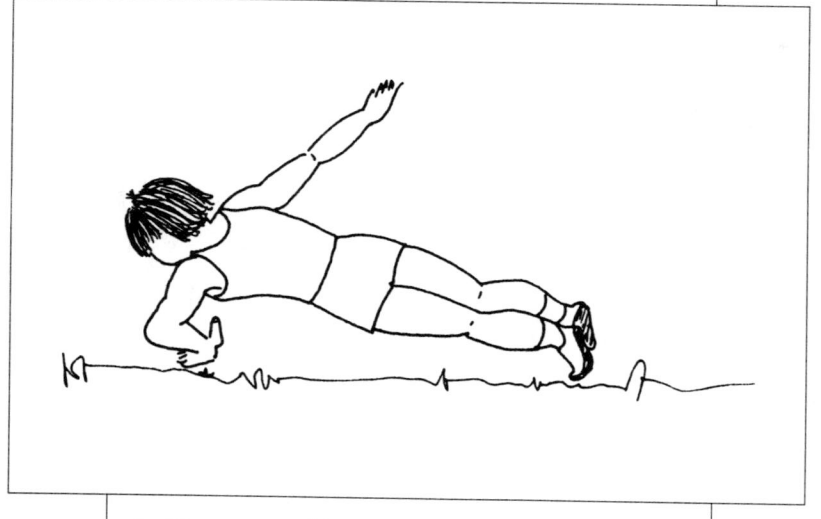

In the tummy position, stretch one arm sideways, while the other one is at chest height next to the body. The bent arm straightens and lifts the body; shift the body weight to the other arm, and move body back to starting position.

General Conditioning

Exercise No. 20

Strengthening Torso Muscles

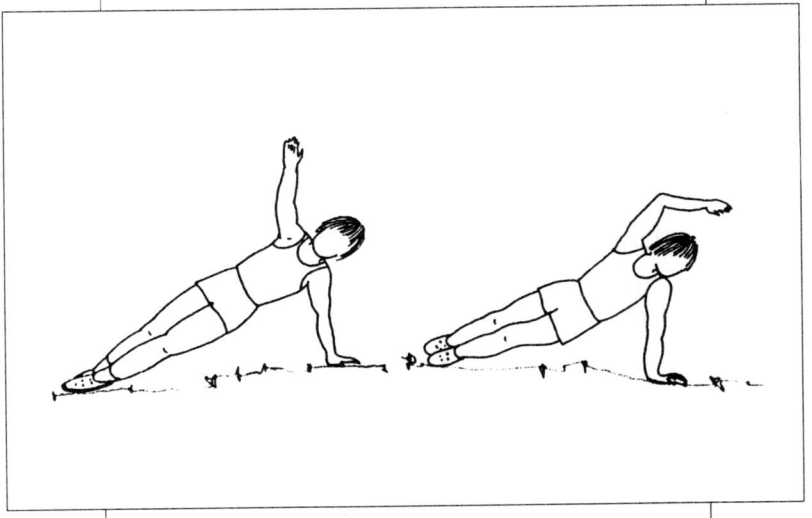

Sideways push-ups, with stretched and bent hip; practice on both sides.

General Conditioning

Exercise No. 21

Strengthening Shoulder Muscles

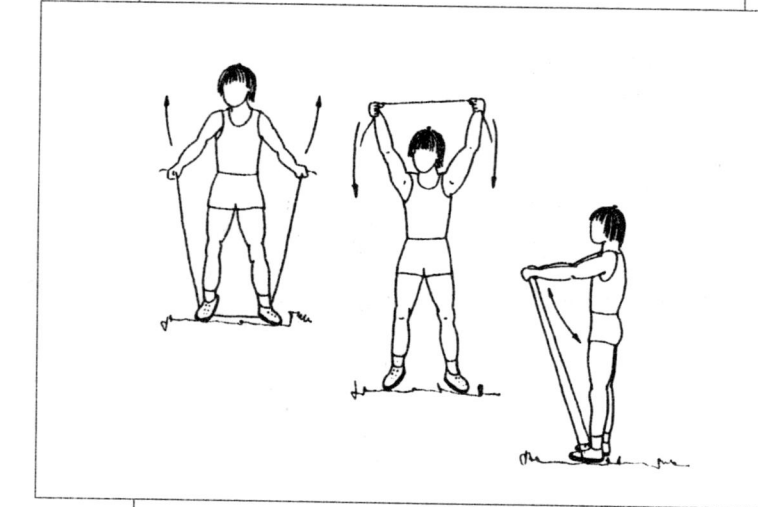

Stand in straddling position on a bicycle innertube, with arms stretched down and holding both ends. Lift and lower arms. Stand with arms overhead holding both ends, and circle arms to the side. Stand in the first position again with the innertube held in front. Lift and lower stretched arms.

General Conditioning

Exercise No. 22

Strengthening Upper Arm Muscles

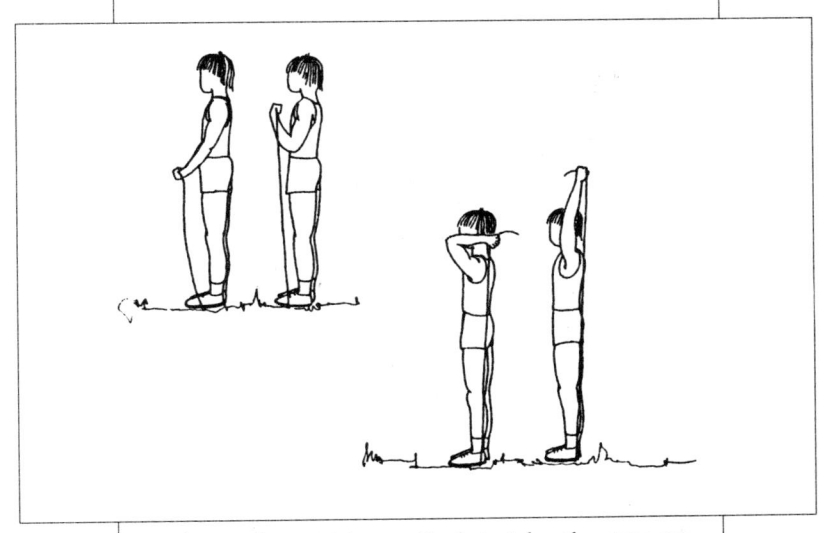

In the starting position on the innertube, the arms are down with each hand holding one end. Bend and stretch arms from the elbow joint. Then, from the same starting position, hold one end of the tube in each hand behind the head and stretch arms up and down.

General Conditioning

Exercise No. 23

Strengthening Upper Arms, Shoulder and Stomach Muscles

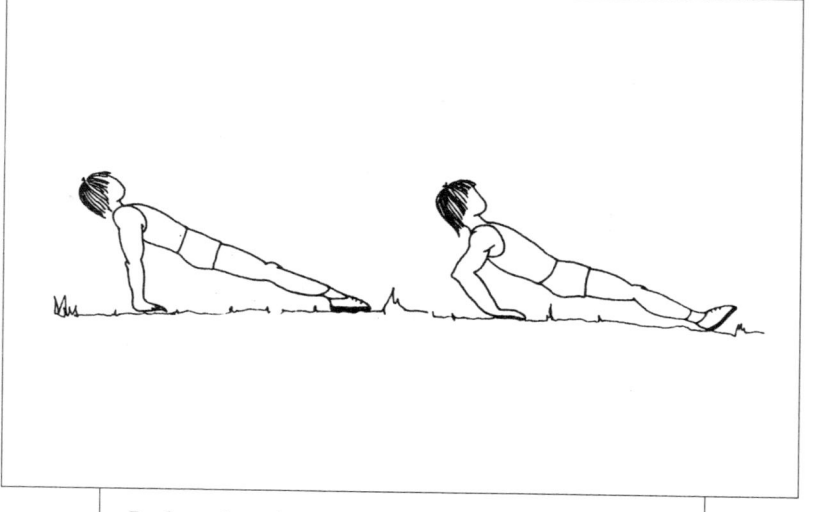

Backwards push-ups: bend the arms and lower the body as much as possible, then straighten arms again and return to starting position.

General Conditioning

Exercise No. 24

Strengthening the Stretching Muscles of the Arms

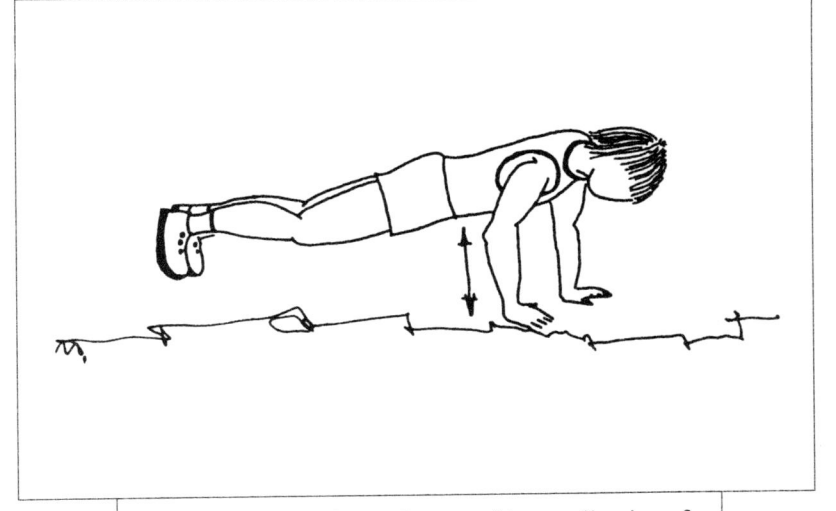

Push-ups: bend and stretch arms with no collapsing of hips! In addition, while pushing up, try to alternately lift feet off the floor while clapping your hands.

General Conditioning

Exercise No. 25

Strengthening Leg Muscles and Improving Coordination

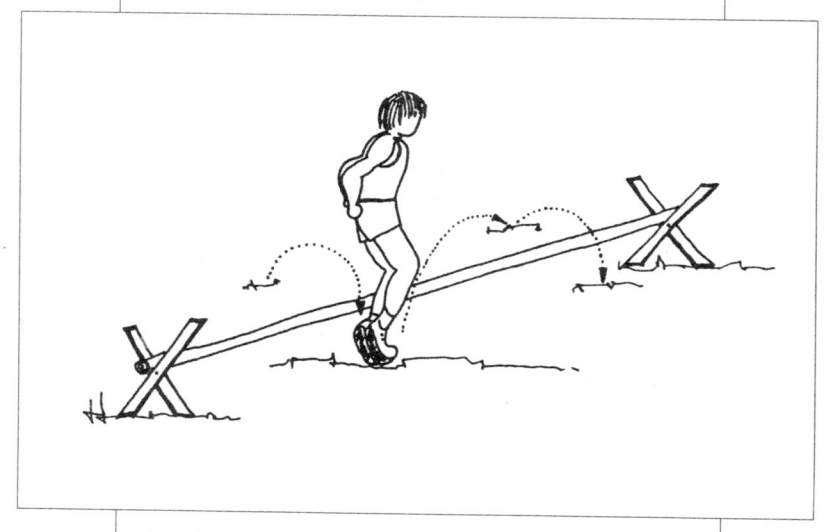

Jumping with feet close together over cavalettis. Try from both sides.

General Conditioning

Exercise No. 26

Strengthening Stomach, Shoulder, and Arm Muscles

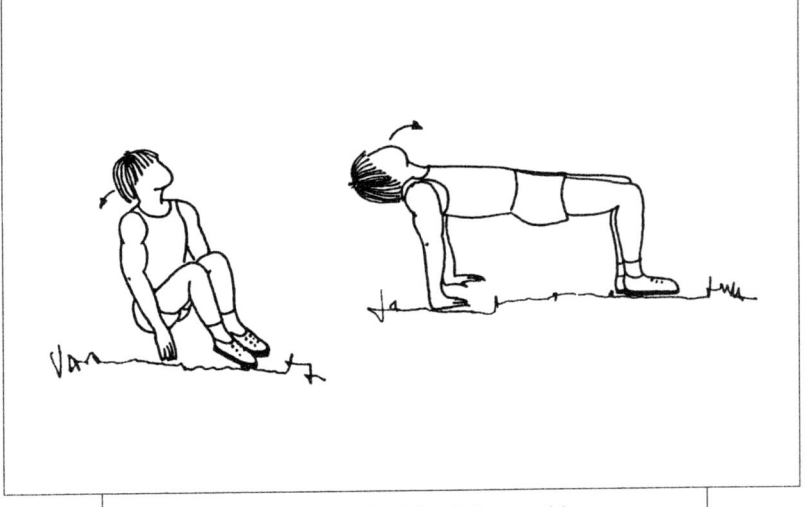

Raise and lower the head while sitting, and in a reverse push-up position with bent lower legs.

General Conditioning

Exercise No. 27

Strengthening Arm, Shoulder, Stomach, and Back Muscles

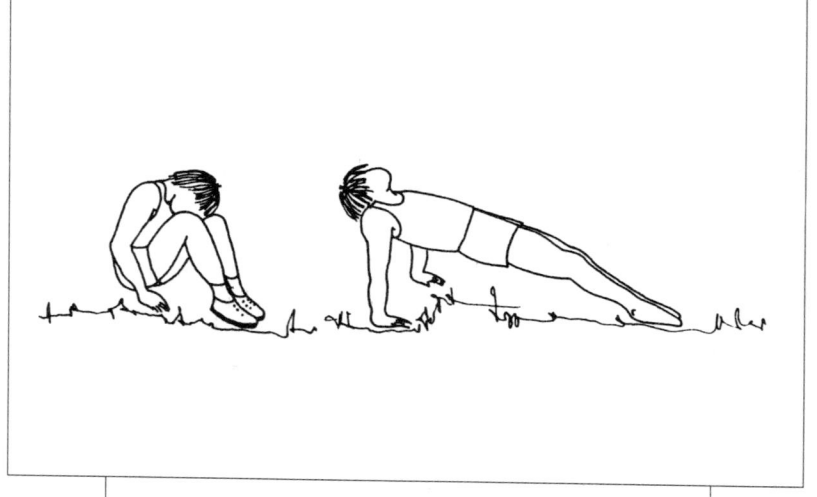

Move from a squatting seat to push-up position alternately.

General Conditioning

Exercise No. 28

Strengthening Stomach Muscles

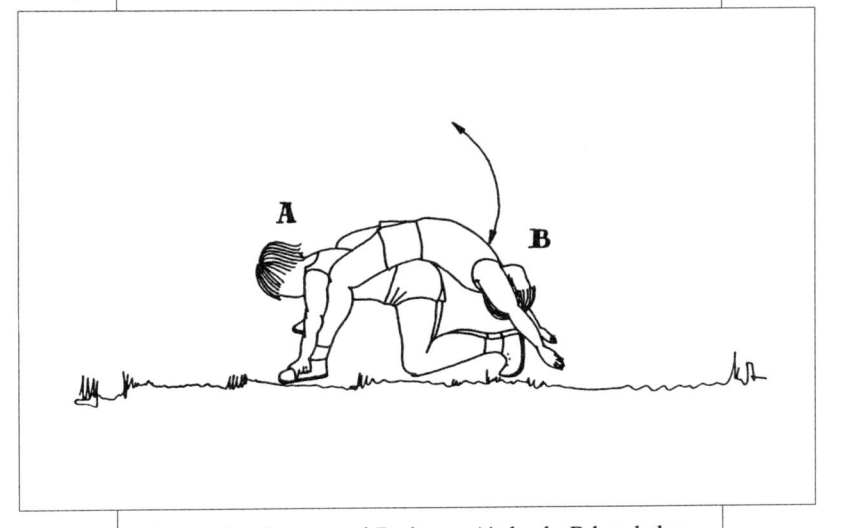

A is on her knees, and B sits on A's back. B bends her upper body backwards and then sits up again, while A holds B's feet down.

Practical Part I

General Conditioning Stretching Exercises

General Conditioning

Exercise No. 29

Stretching Shoulder Muscles

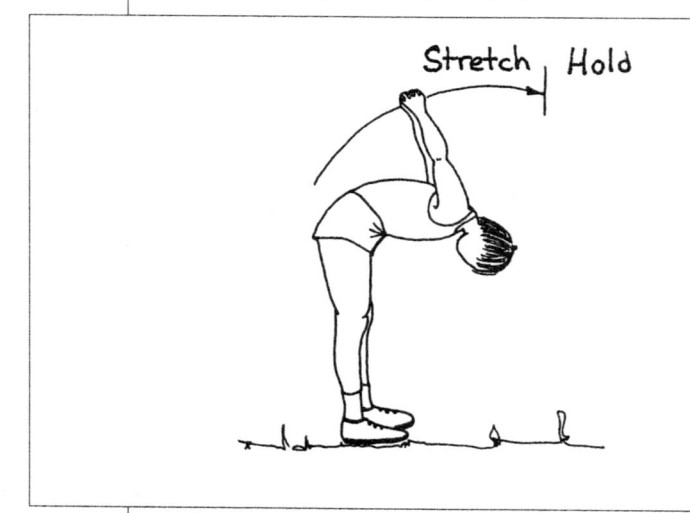

Bending the upper body, spring arms forward in the direction of the arrow several times and hold a few seconds.

General Conditioning

Exercise No. 30

Stretching the Back of the Thigh

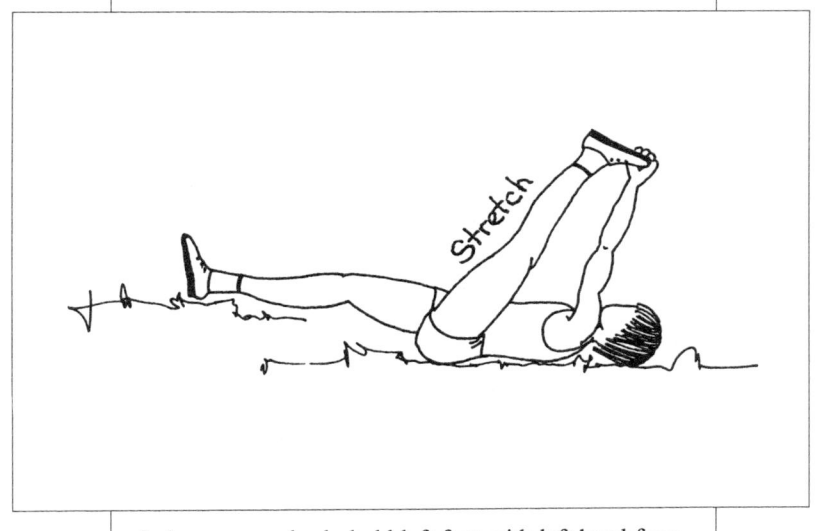

Lying on your back, hold left foot with left hand from inside, stretch leg, and hold.

General Conditioning

Exercise No. 31

Stretching the Front of the Body

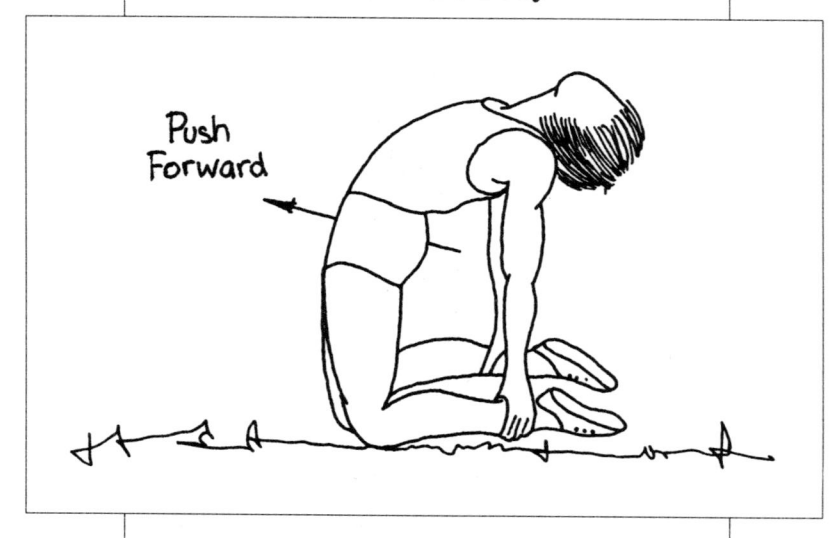

Push Forward

On your knees, with upper body upright, hold ankles and push pelvis forward.

General Conditioning

Exercise No. 32

Stretching the Body Muscles

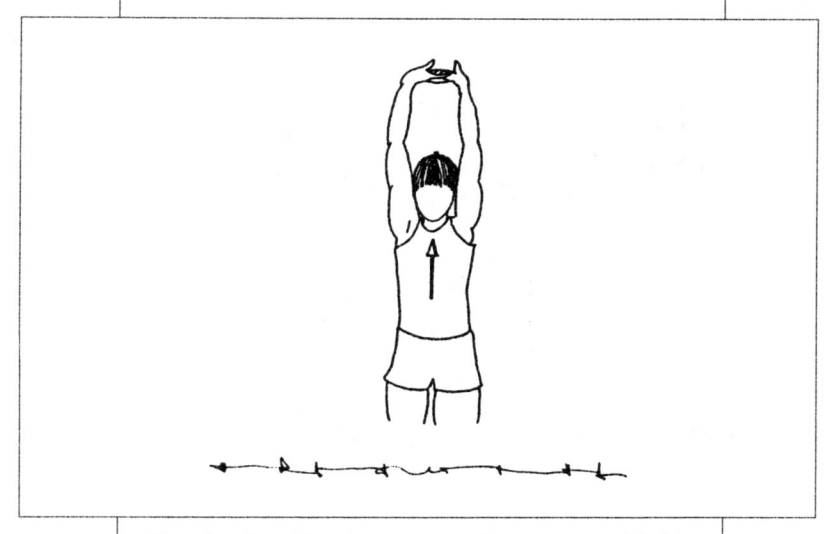

Clasp hands with palms up, stretch torso up and hold.

General Conditioning

Exercise No. 33

Stretching the Body Muscles

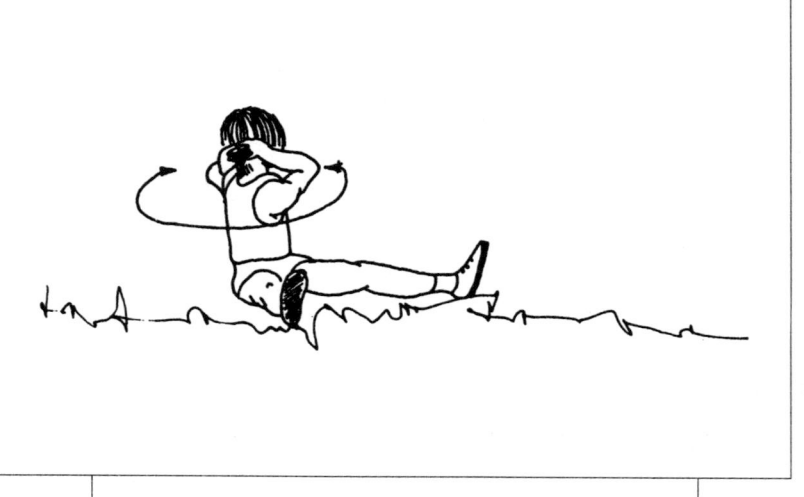

The Torso Twist: sit on the floor with legs apart and turn body vigorously to both sides.

General Conditioning

Exercise No. 34

Stretching the Back of the Thighs

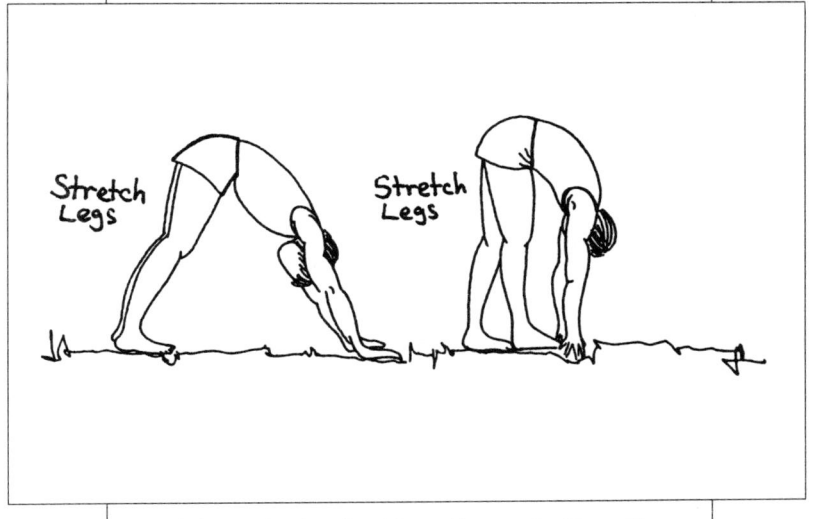

Walk forward to hands with totally stretched legs. Keep your fingers on the floor.

General Conditioning

Exercise No. 35

Stretching the Back of the Thighs

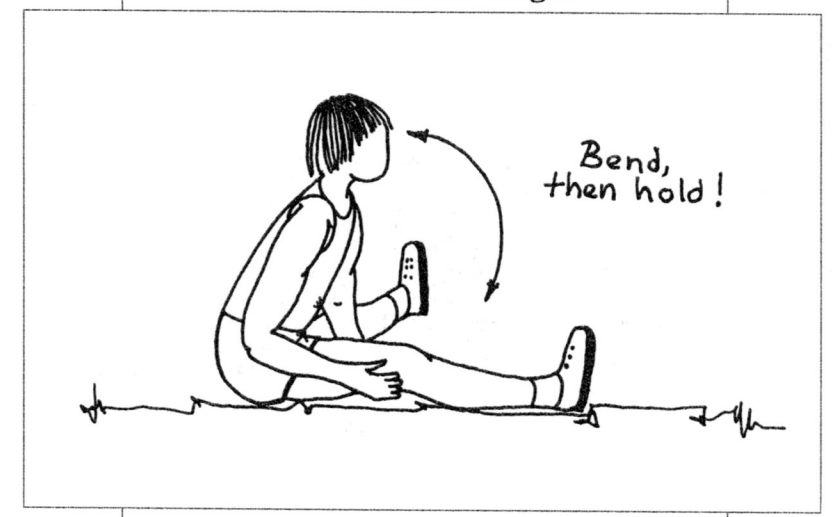

Bend, then hold!

Bow with straightened upper body over right, then left leg. Stretch toward the floor a few times over each leg, and hold.

General Conditioning

Exercise No. 36

Stretching the Back of Thighs and Back Muscles

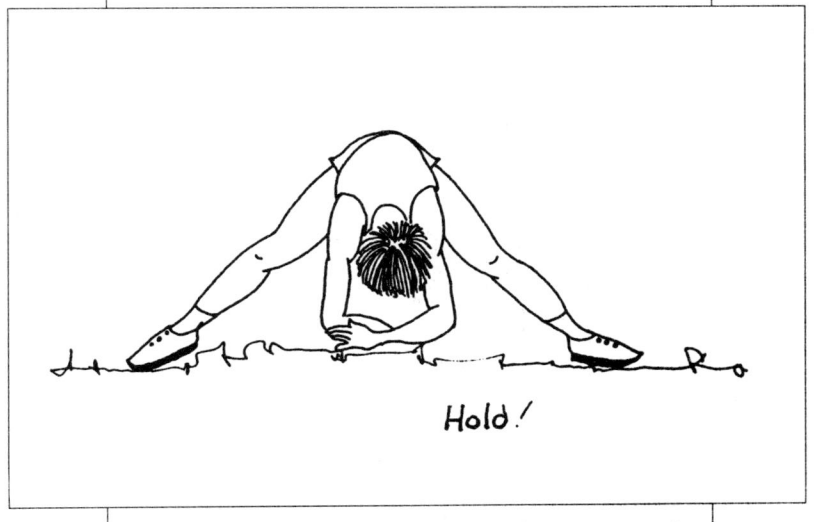

Hold!

Straddle your legs with locked knees; lower arms, and touch the floor. Stretch toward floor and hold.

General Conditioning

Exercise No. 37

Stretching the Front of Thighs and Flexors of Hips

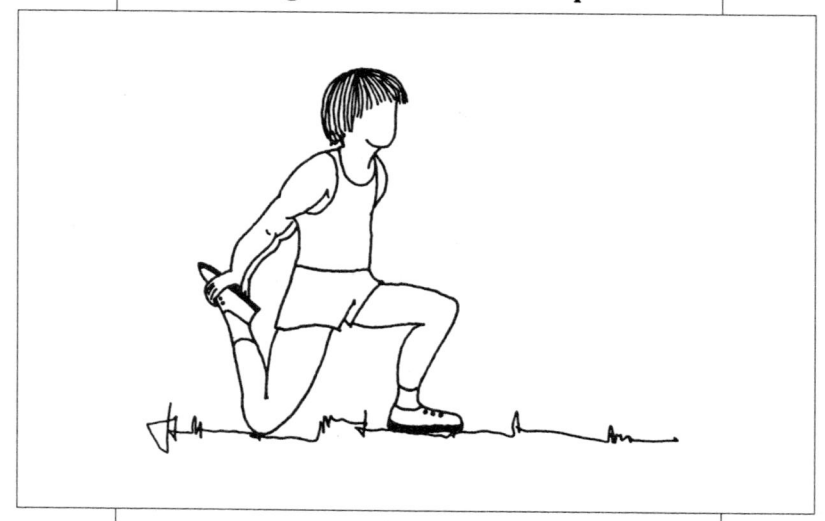

Pull your foot up to your seat, first with one hand, then with both.

General Conditioning

Exercise No. 38

Stretching of Torso and Hip Muscles, Increasing Mobility of Hips and Shoulder Joints

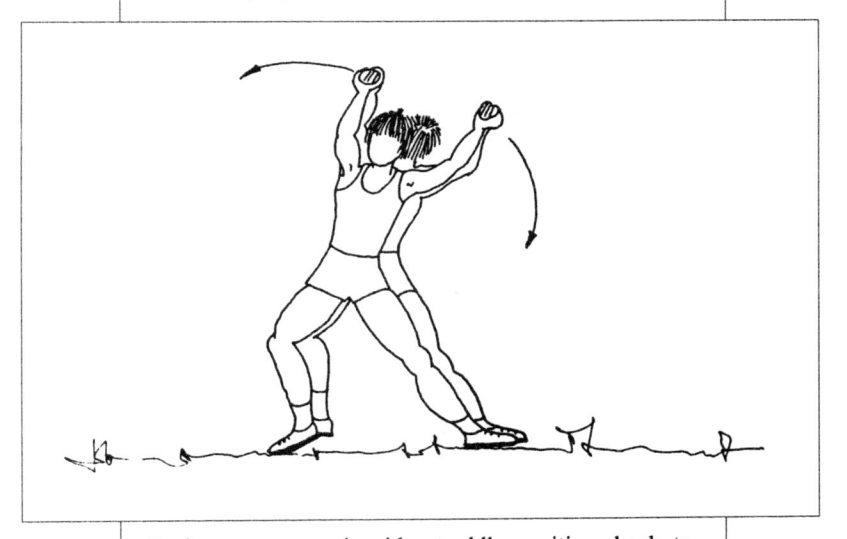

Both partners are in side straddle position, back to back, with arms up and hands held. Step aside together with one leg and bend stretched upper body towards stretched leg.

General Conditioning

Exercise No. 39

Stretching of Back Muscles and Back of Thighs

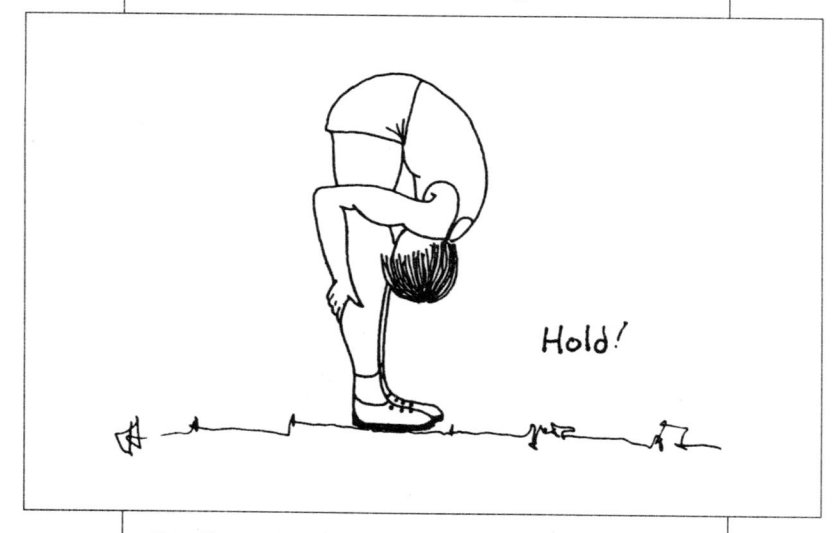

Standing, pull your head towards stretched legs (knees), hold!

General Conditioning

Exercise No. 40

Stretching the Front of Thighs, Back and Seat Muscles

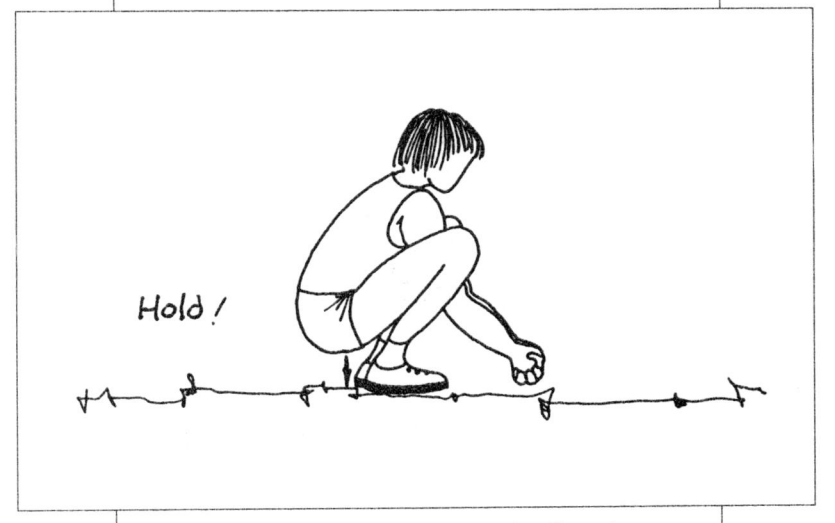

Hold!

The squatting vault: with heels on the floor, bounce, then hold.

Practical Part I

General Conditioning

Flexibility Exercises

General Conditioning

Exercise No. 41

Mobility of the Spine

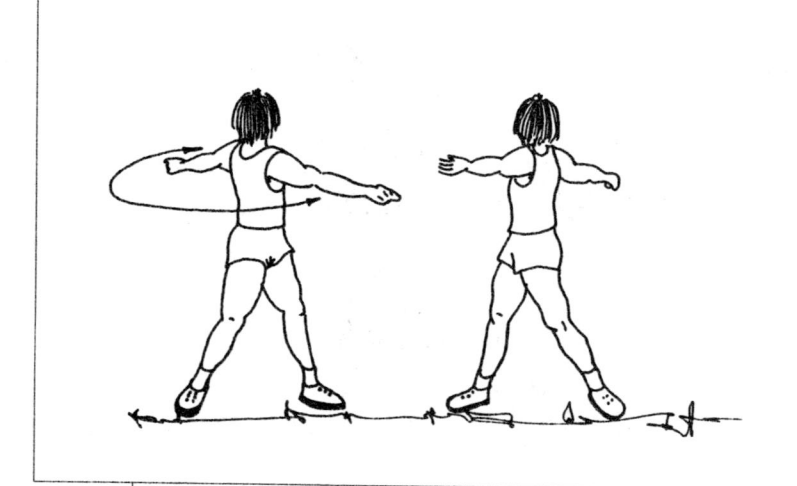

Turning torso: arms swing loosely around the body. *Do not* lift heels.

General Conditioning

Exercise No. 42

Mobility of the Spine

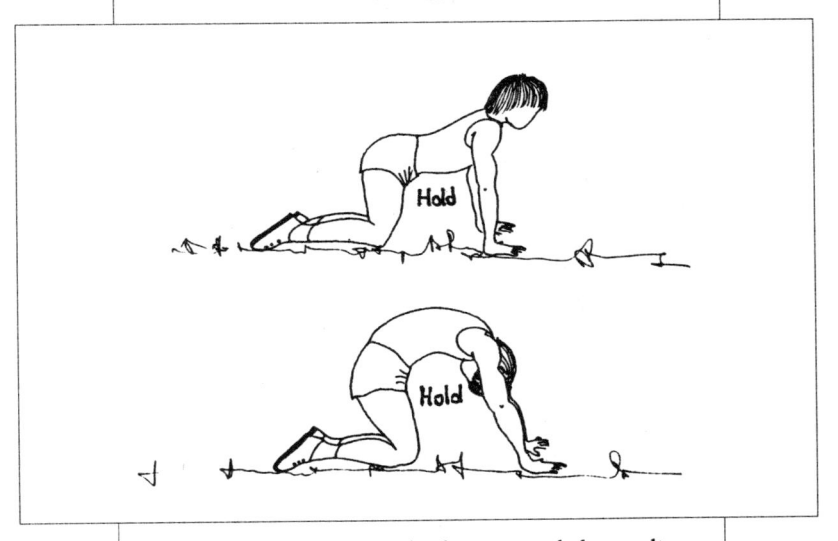

On hands and knees, push chest up and down alternately. Hold at highest and lowest points.

General Conditioning

Exercise No. 43

Mobility of the Spine

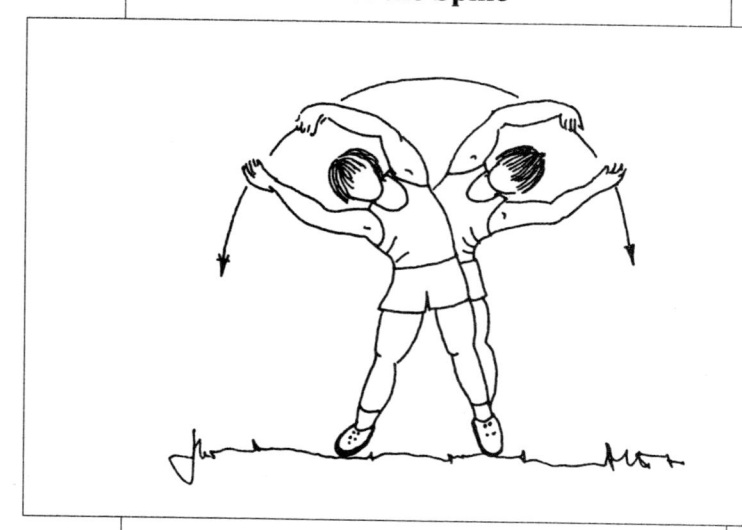

Bend the torso sideways: hold arms up, bend upper body to right and left. The body stays stretched, and hips do not move forward or back.

General Conditioning

Exercise No. 44

Mobility of the Upper Chest

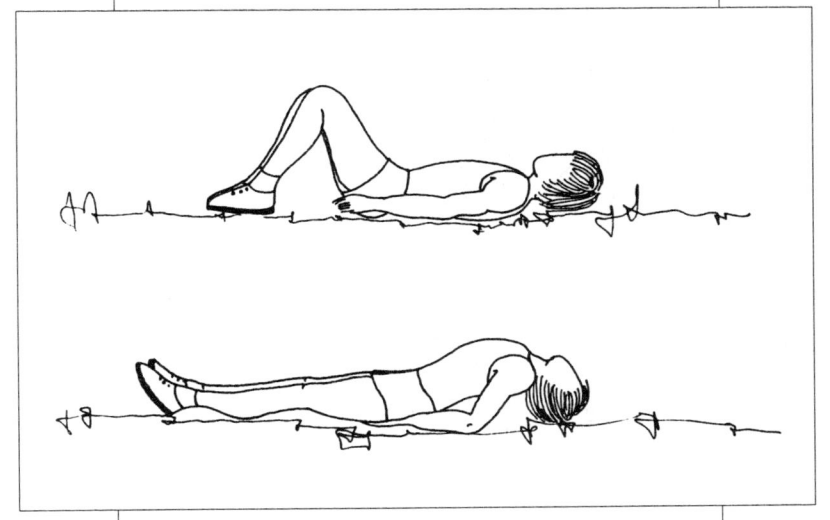

Picture 1: Lie flat on your back and pull legs up.
Picture 2: Stretch legs out, and bend neck backwards. Lift chest at the same time, hold for a moment.

General Conditioning

Exercise No. 45

Mobility of Pelvis, and Stretching the Front of the Thigh

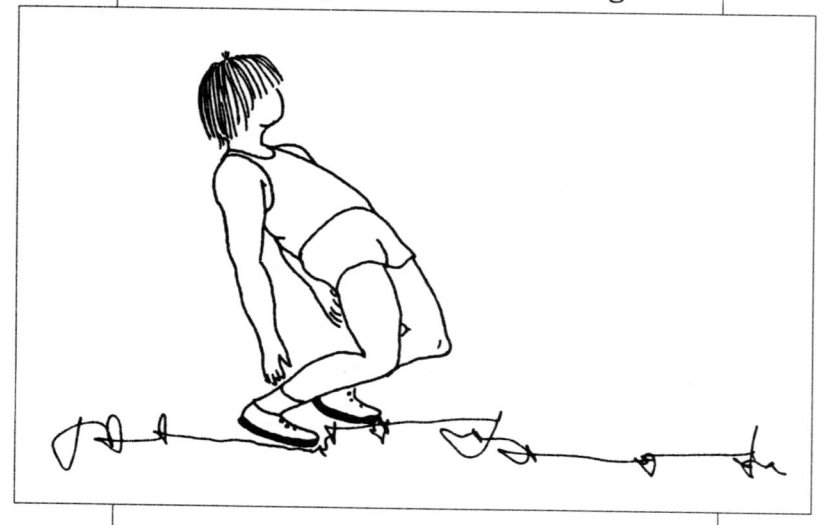

With your torso bending backwards, touch your ankles with both hands, with slightly straddled legs. Keep your pelvis forward and in front.

General Conditioning

Exercise No. 46

Mobility of Spine and Pelvic Region

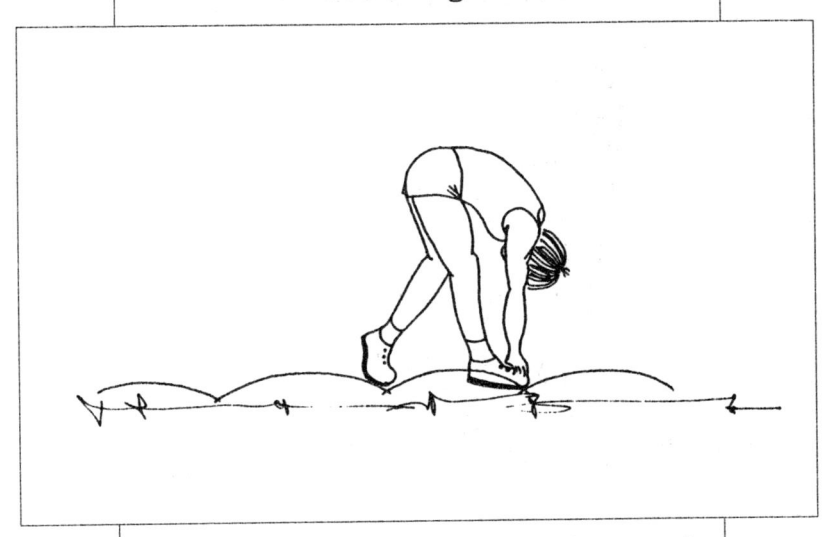

Torso elasticity: walk forward with small steps, and "be elastic" over the forward leg.

General Conditioning

Exercise No. 47

Mobility of the Spine

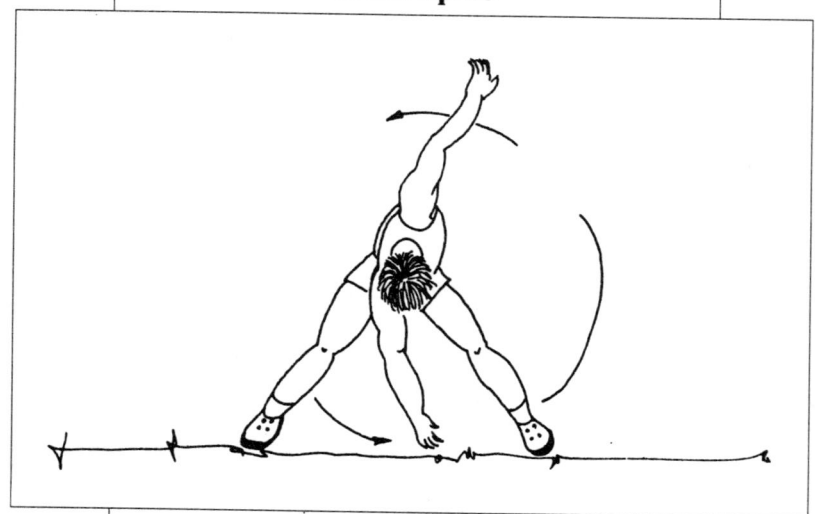

Torso-turn with flexion forward: the left hand touches right foot, and the right hand touches left foot. Keep legs stretched!

General Conditioning

Exercise No. 48

Mobility of Hips and Lower Back;
Stretching the back of thighs, while bending back, stretch stomach and hip muscles.

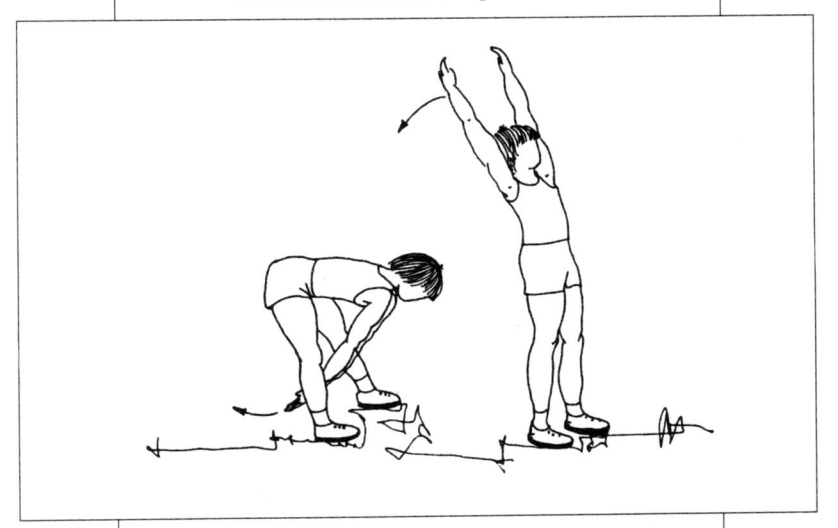

In the straddle position with arms up, bend the upper body forward. Try to touch the floor between your legs with your hands, then arms up again and bend your upper body back.

General Conditioning

Exercise No. 49

Mobility of the Spine, Strengthening of Arm and Shoulder Muscles

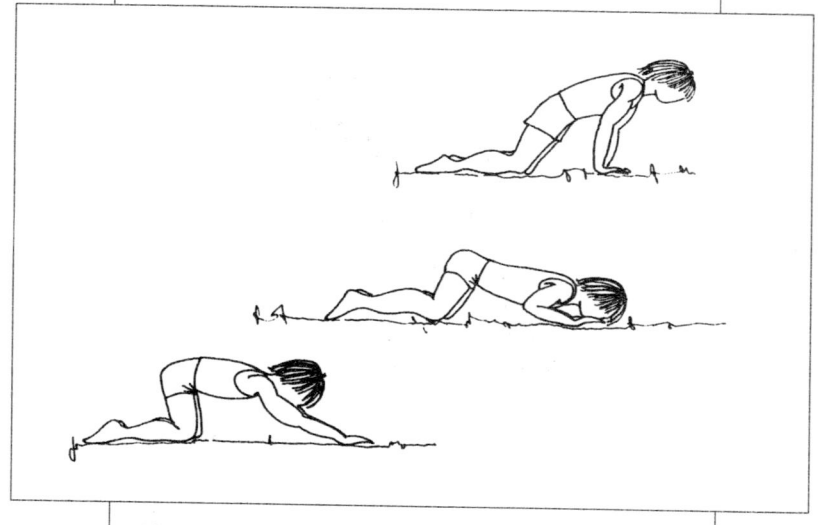

The kneestand: bend the upper body forward. Hands touch the floor with straightened arms, then bend arms and chest as deeply as possible towards floor while bringing your upper body forward. Then straighten arms again, round your back and return to the starting position.

General Conditioning

Exercise No. 50

Flexibility of Shoulder Joints, Stretching of Shoulders and Chest Muscles

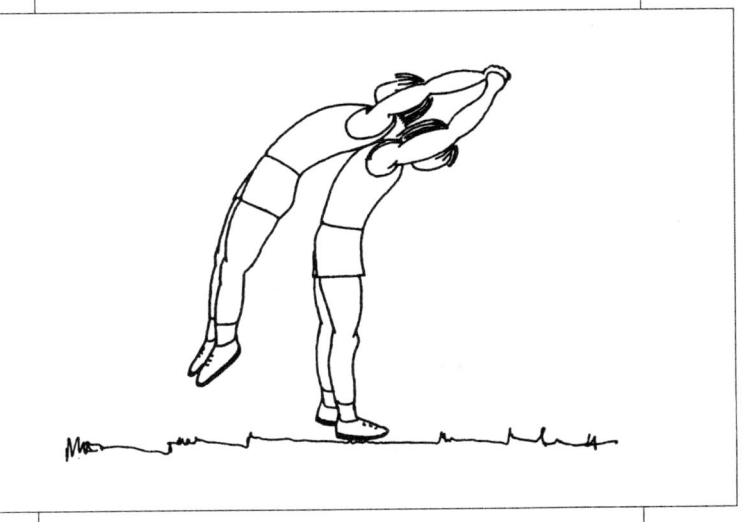

Both partners are in the side straddle position, back to back, with arms up and hands held. A bends her upper body forward and carries B only on her shoulders—lower backs do not touch.

Practical Part I

General Conditioning

Coordination Exercises

General Conditioning

Exercise No. 51

Coordination and Strengthening the Leg Muscles

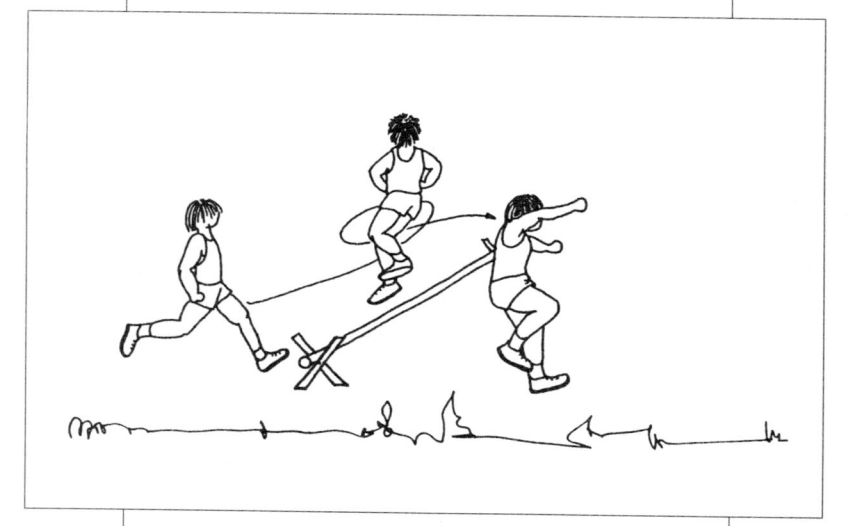

Leap in a pivoting motion over cavalettis, turning to both sides.

General Conditioning

Exercise No. 52

Coordination and General Conditioning

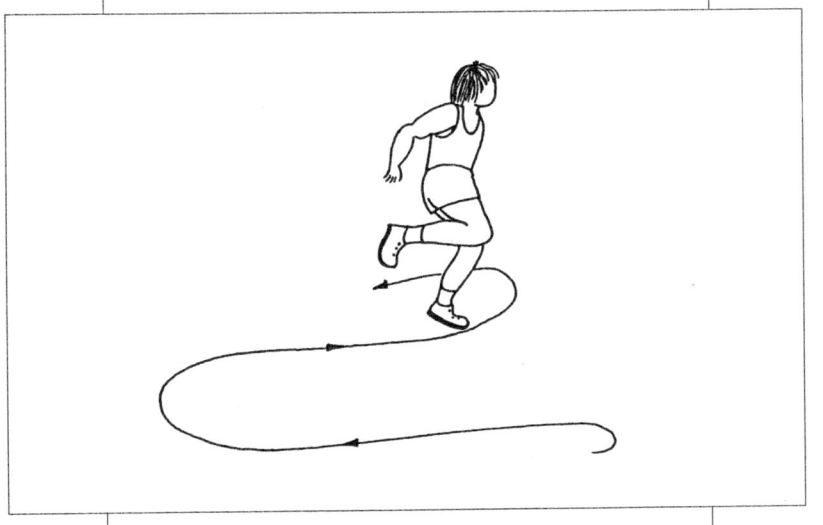

Jog on curved lines through the arena, using different tempos.

General Conditioning

Exercise No. 53

Coordination, Strengthening of Shoulder, Hip, and Leg Muscles

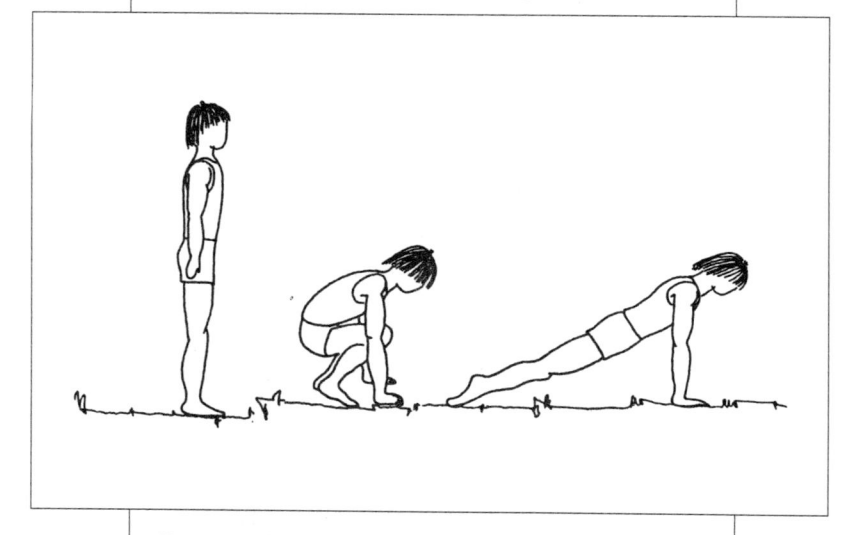

From starting position to squatting position, then to push-up position. Bend arms and lower body to the floor. Then straighten arms again, jump back to squatting position and return to starting.

General Conditioning

Exercise No. 54

Coordination and Strengthening the Leg Muscles

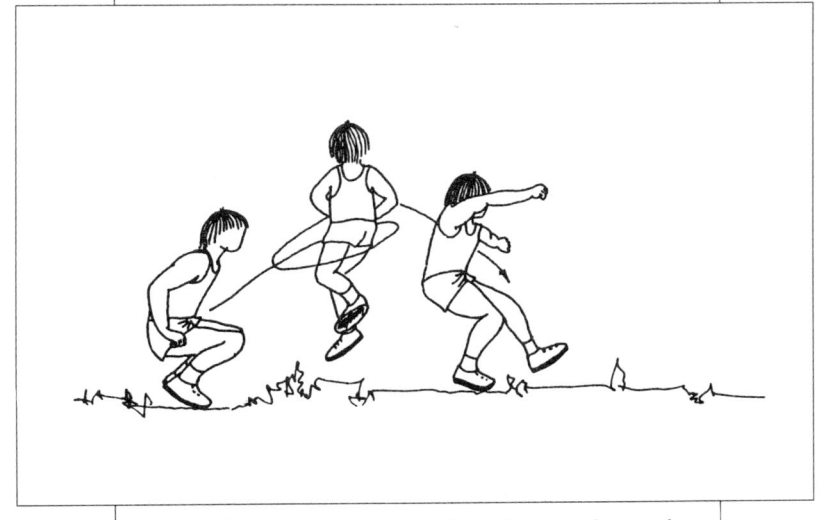

Turning jumps with both legs from the squatting vault: from a deep squatting position, vault back into a deep squatting position. **Note:** Turn during the jump, totally stretching in the air for a moment.

General Conditioning

Exercise No. 55

Coordination and Strengthening the Leg Muscles

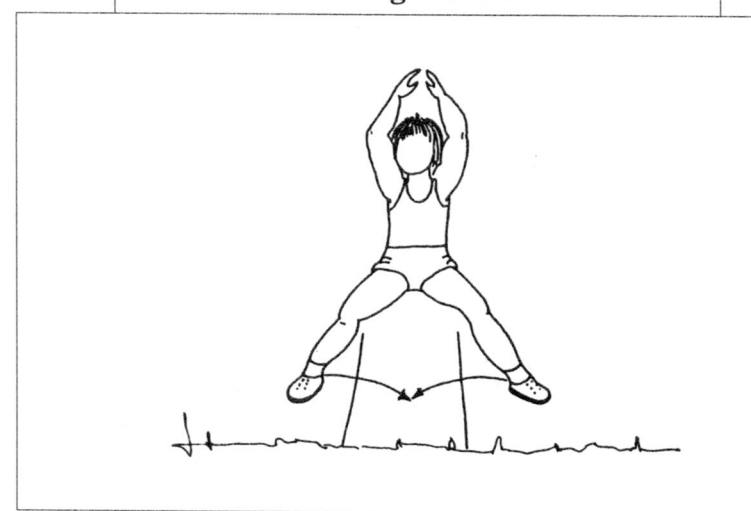

Jumping Jack: jump from feet together to spreading legs, while clapping hands above the head. Jump back immediately, with hands touching legs.

General Conditioning

Exercise No. 56

Coordination and Strengthening the Leg Muscles

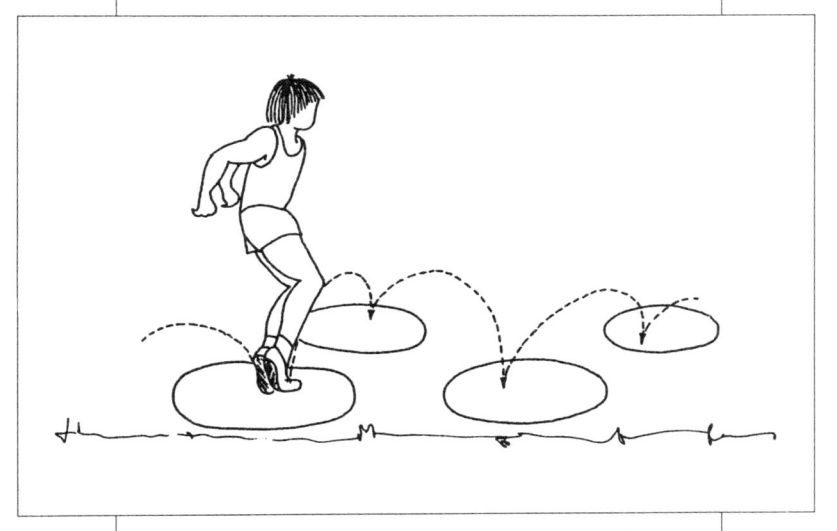

Circle jumping with both feet: jump from circle to circle with feet together, first with a jump in between, then without.

General Conditioning

Exercise No. 57

Coordination, Stimulation of Cardiovascular System

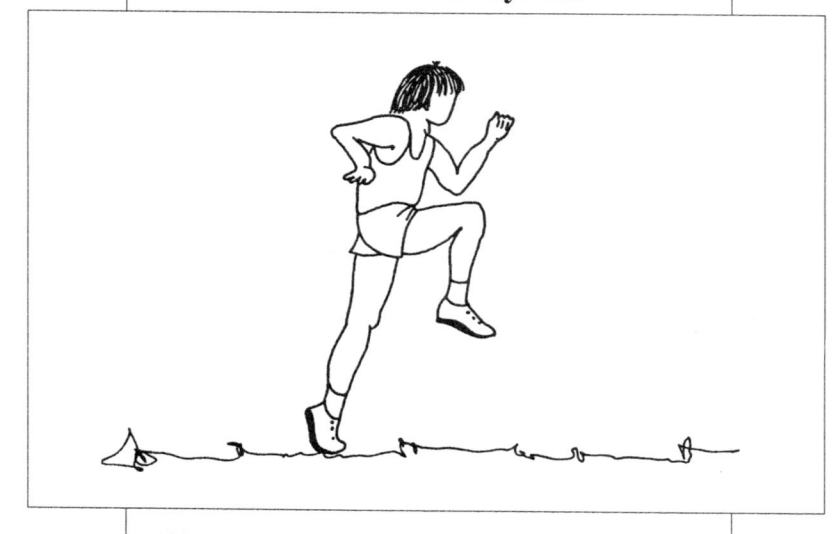

Skipping in place or traveling: step quickly, bringing knees to a horizontal position. Swing arms the same as in normal jogging, do not tense.

General Conditioning

Exercise No. 58

Coordination and Strengthening the Leg Muscles

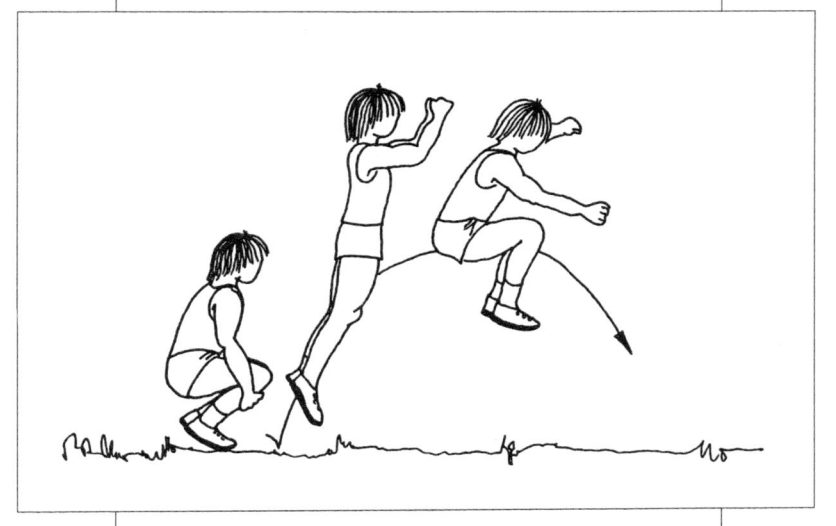

Jump from a deep squatting crouch, lifting knees to the chest.

General Conditioning

Exercise No. 59

Coordination and Strengthening the Leg Muscles

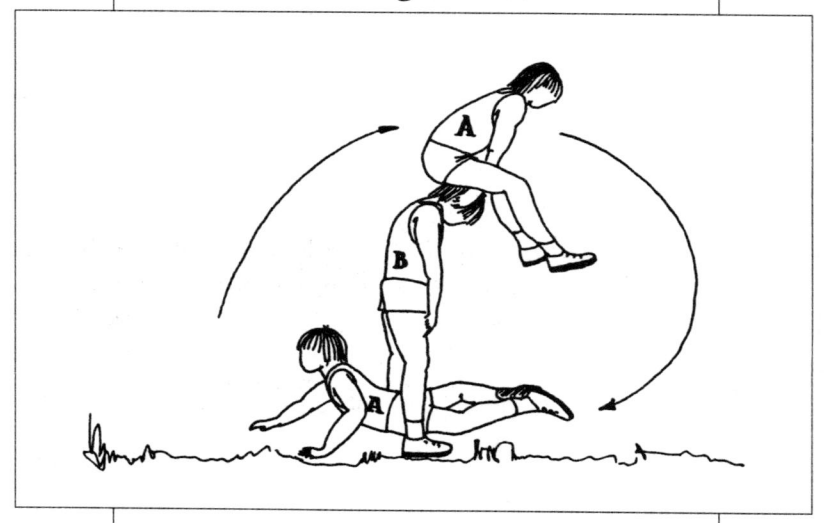

Partner A leapfrogs over B, then crawls back through the legs of B.

Practical Part II

Additional Exercises for Riders

Strengthening Exercises

Additional Exercises for Riders

Exercise No. 60

Coordination and Strengthening of Leg Muscles

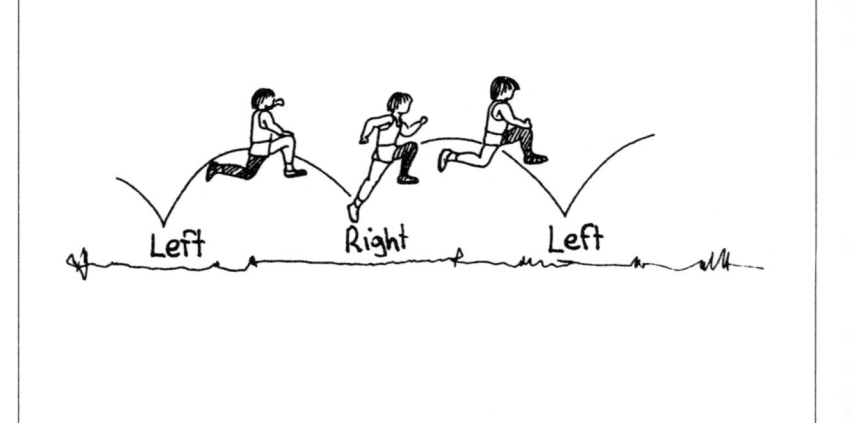

While skipping, raise thighs to horizontal position. When left leg is in the air, the right arm should be forward and up. **Note:** Gain as much ground as possible.

Additional Exercises for Riders

Exercise No. 61

Strengthening of Back Muscles
(especially the lower seat muscles)

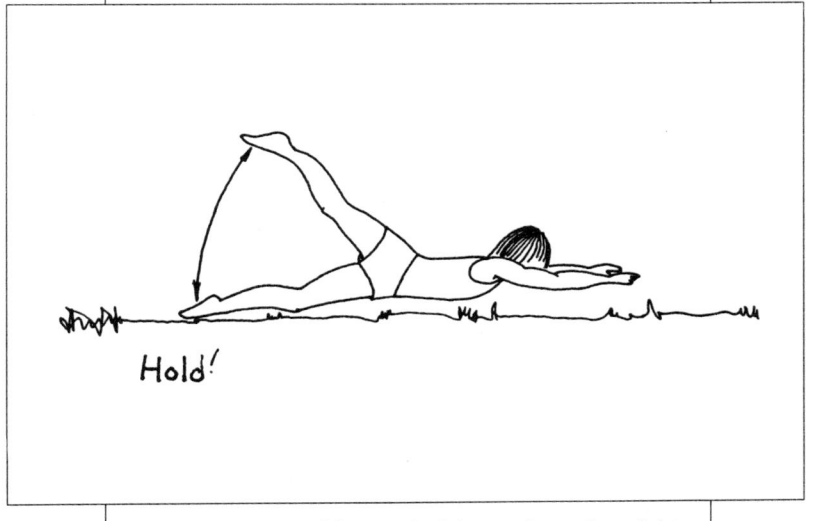

Hold!

On your tummy, lift stretched legs, alternating right and left and hold for a moment in the highest position.

Additional Exercises for Riders

Exercise No. 62

Strengthening Stomach And Hip Muscles

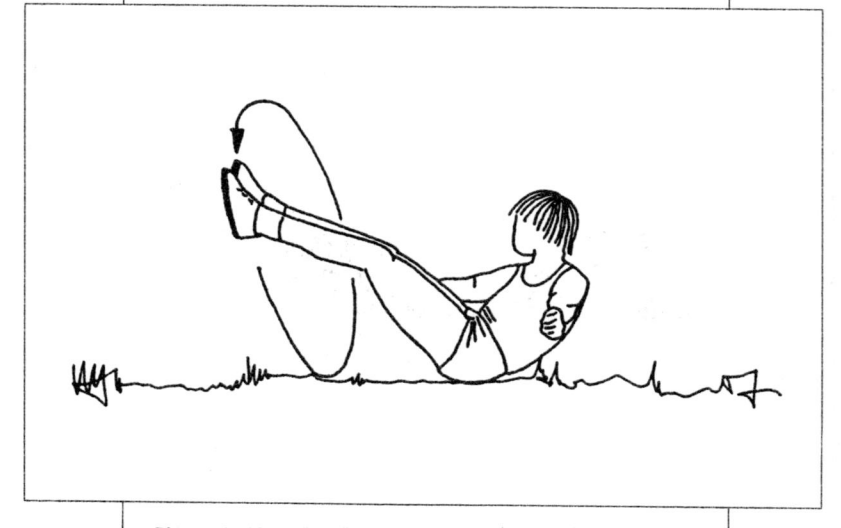

Sit on the floor, with arms up, and circle closed straight legs in both directions.

Additional Exercises for Riders

Exercise No. 63

Strengthening Back and Seat Muscles

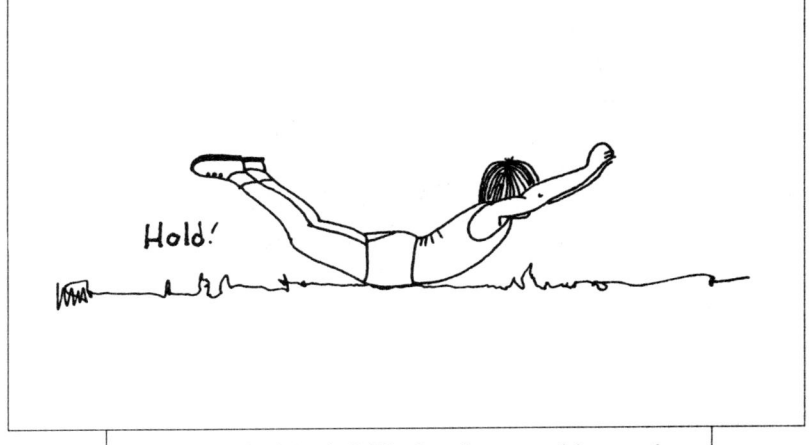

Hold!

The "Stretched Scale." lift closed arms and legs at the same time, hold for a moment.

Additional Exercises for Riders

Exercise No. 64

Strengthening Calves

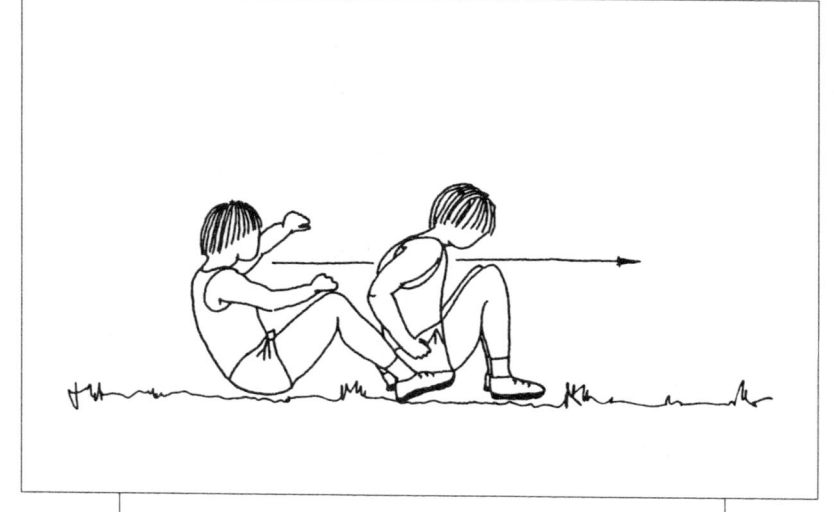

Sit on the floor, with arms up, and pull seat to heels.

Additional Exercises for Riders

Exercise No. 65

Strengthening Thigh Muscles

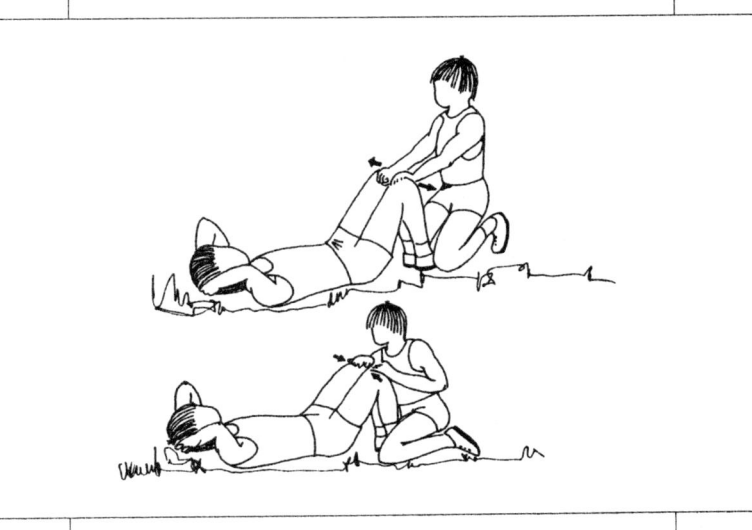

A lies on her back with legs bent. B tries to pull A's knees apart. Then A opens knees slightly, and B tries to push them together.

Additional Exercises for Riders

Exercise No. 65

Strengthening Leg Muscles (Inside/Outside)

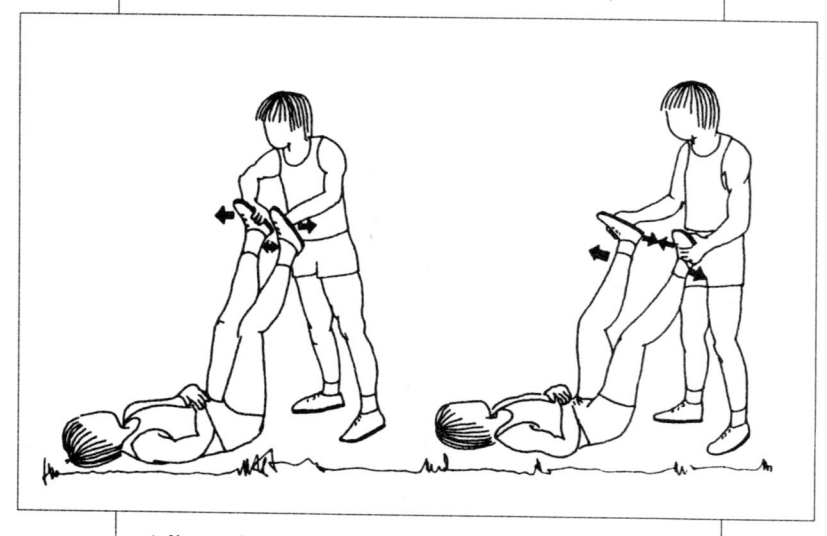

A lies on her back with legs extended and closed. B tries to pull them apart. Then A holds her legs open and B tries to push them together.

Additional Exercises for Riders

Exercise No. 67

Strengthening Stomach and Hip Muscles

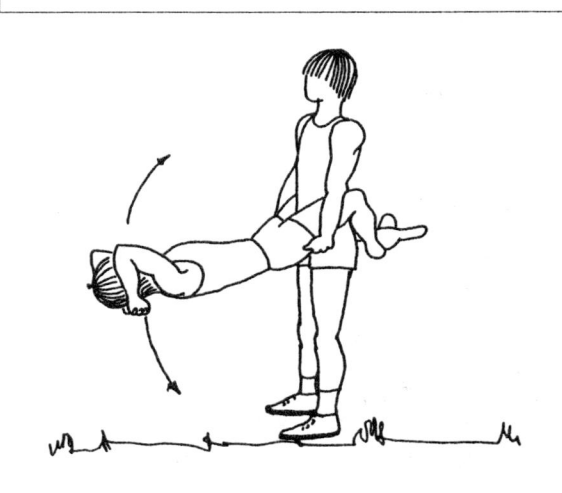

A stands, legs apart. B sits on the hips of A with her legs folded behind A's back, and hands behind her neck. B then bends her upper body forward and back.

Additional Exercises for Riders

Exercise No. 68

Strengthening Stomach Muscles

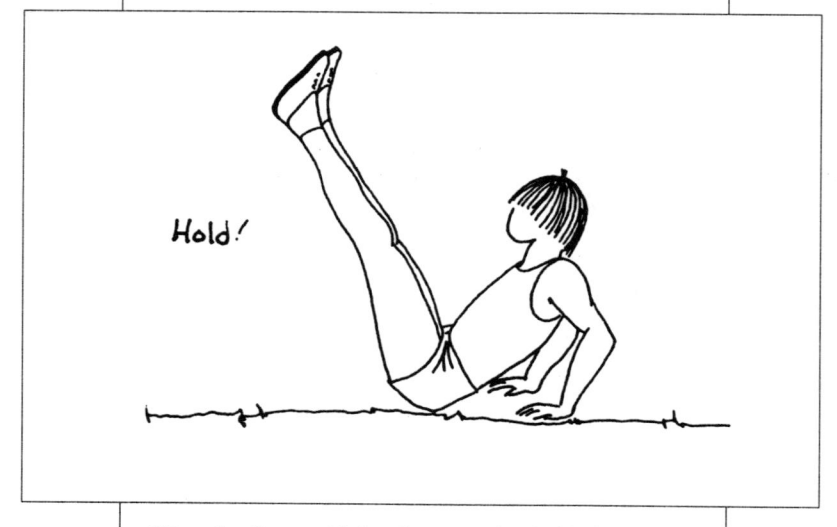

Hold!

Sit on the floor, with hands supporting behind you. Lift stretched legs and hold for a moment.

Additional Exercises for Riders

Exercise No. 69

Strengthening Back, Leg, and Hip Muscles

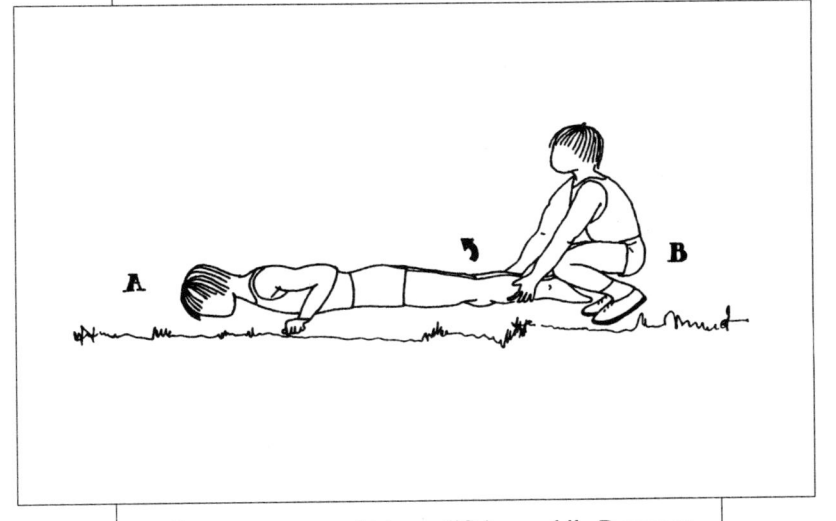

A lies on tummy, and tries to lift legs, while B presses them down.

Additional Exercises for Riders

Exercise No. 70

Strengthening Back, Torso, Hip, and Shoulder Muscles

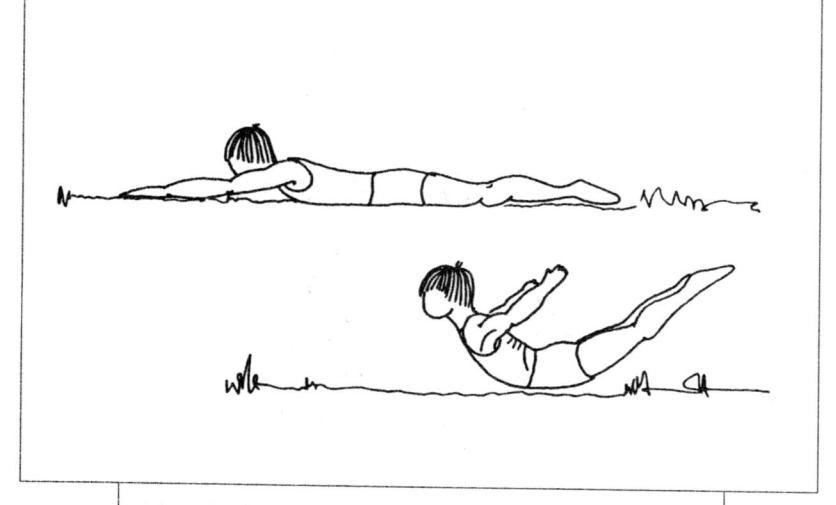

On your tummy with arms extended over the head, lift your upper body while holding arms to the side. Lift stretched legs, and rock longitudinally in this position, then return to starting position.

Additional Exercises for Riders

Exercise No. 71

Strengthening Stomach Muscles

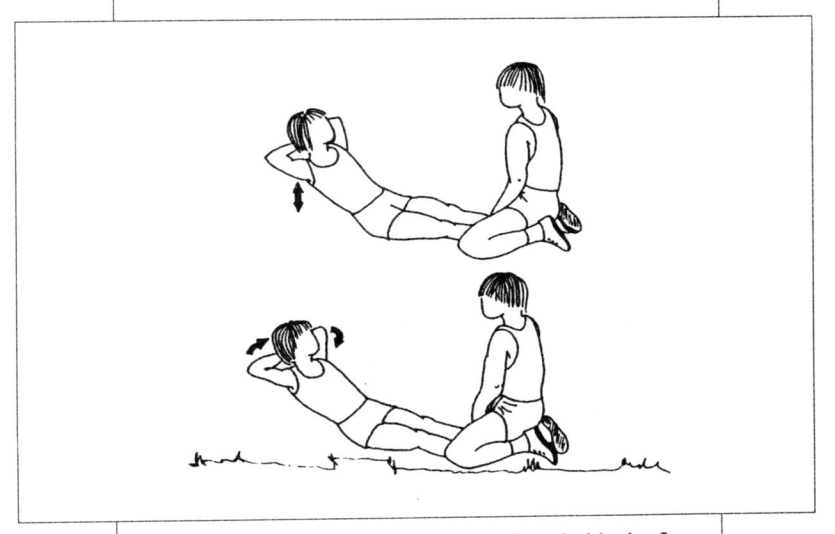

A lies with her back on the floor, while B holds the feet of her stretched legs. A rises up; then repeats and twists her upper body while in the up position.

Additional Exercises for Riders

Exercise No. 72

Strengthening Back Muscles

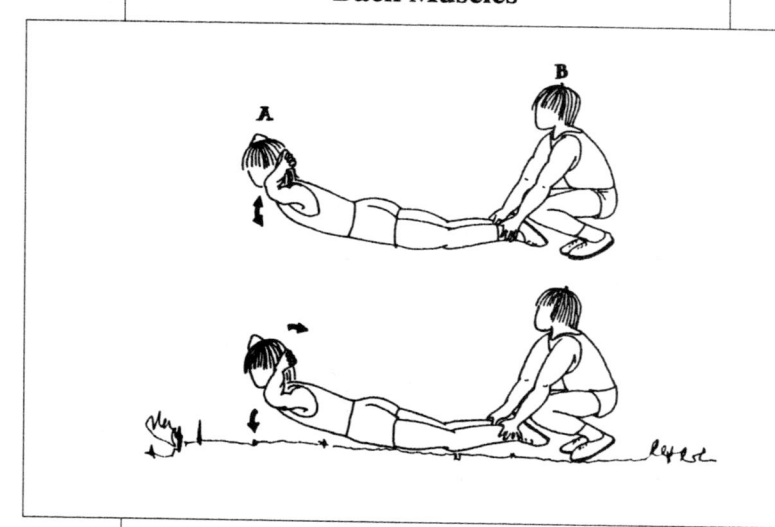

A lies on her stomach, and B holds her legs. A lifts her upper body with arms folded behind her head. Repeat the same exercise, but twist the lifted upper body from right to left.

Practical Part II

Additional Exercises for Riders

Stretching Exercises

Additional Exercises for Riders

Exercise No. 73

Stretching the Lower Back Muscles, Relieving Tension in the Hip Region, Strengthening Stomach Muscles

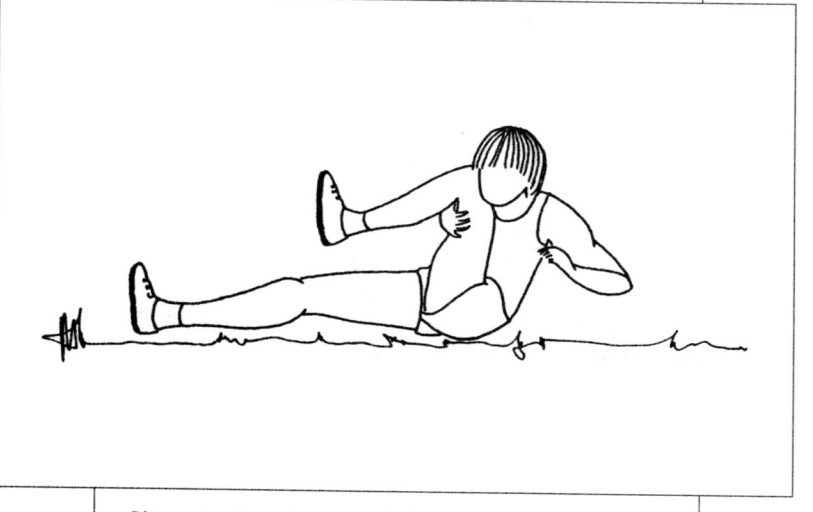

Sit on the floor, and pull left knee with right hand to right shoulder. Hold, then perform the same exercise to the other side.

Additional Exercises for Riders

Exercise No. 74

Stretching the Oblique Torso Muscles, Relieving Tension in the Spinal Region of the Torso and Lower Back.

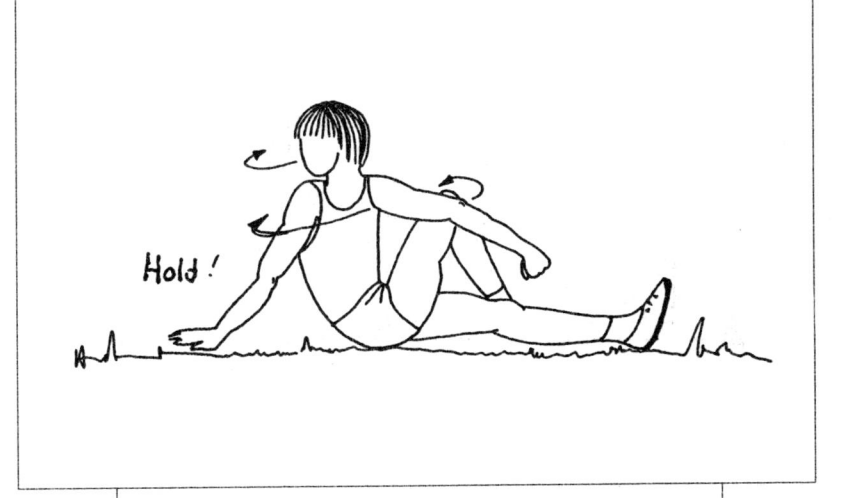

Sit on the floor, and push away right knee using left arm. Turn the torso in the other direction, hold, and then repeat exercise to the other side.

Additional Exercises for Riders

Exercise No. 75

Stretching the Arm Muscles

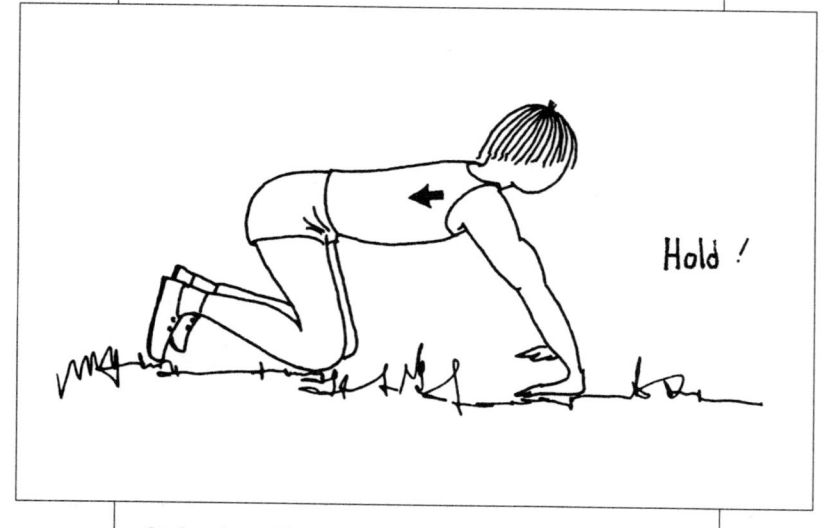

Hold !

On hands and knees, move shoulders back in the direction of the arrow. Fingers point to the knees, hold, then bring your head forward again. If this is difficult in the beginning, start with fingers pointing to the side.

Additional Exercises for Riders

Exercise No. 76

Stretching the Seat Muscles

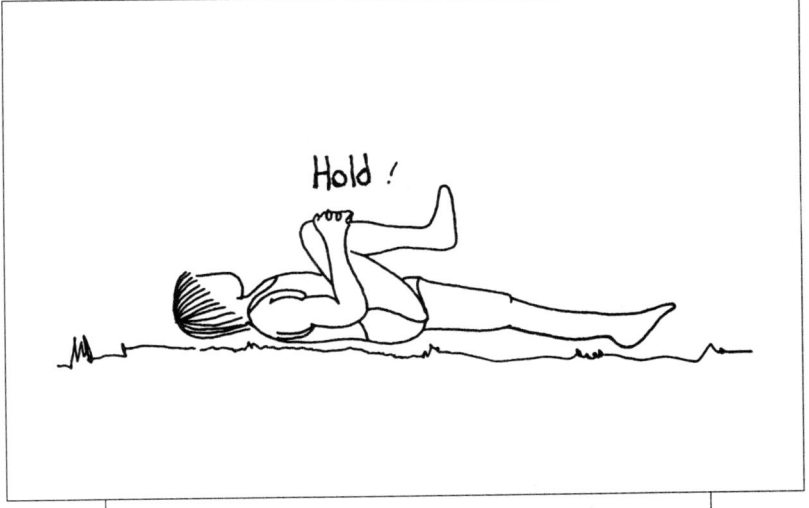

Lie on your back, and pull your knee, right then left, to chest, and hold.

Additional Exercises for Riders

Exercise No. 77

Stretching Front Thigh Muscles and the Muscles Which Bend the Hip

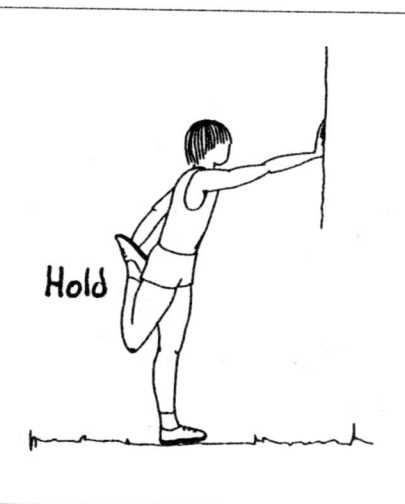

Stand up, and lean against partner or wall. Pull foot up to your seat, and push pelvis forward. Hold. Alternate left and right.

Additional Exercises for Riders

Exercise No. 78

Stretching
Back Thigh Muscles

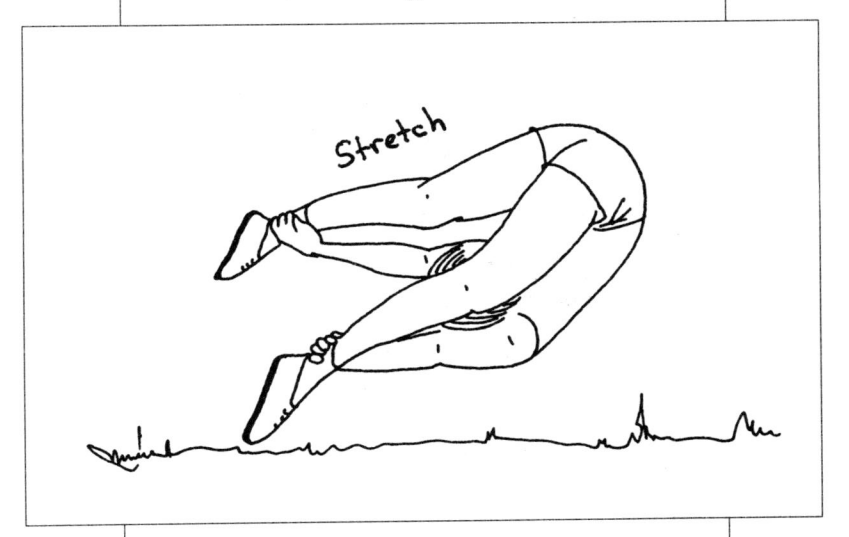

Stretch

Lie on your back with legs straight. Stretch your legs over your head, with hands holding ankles from behind, and pull your feet to the floor. Hold.

Additional Exercises for Riders

Exercise No. 79

Stretching the Front Torso

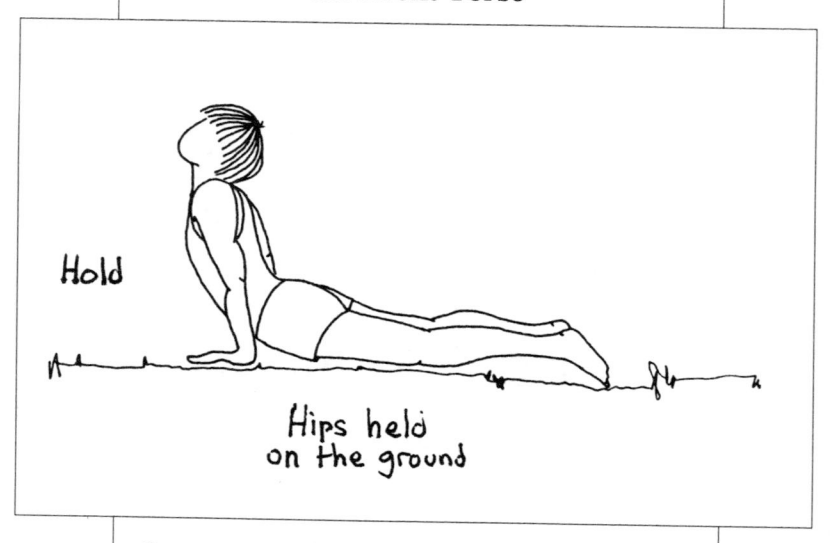

Hold

Hips held on the ground

On your tummy, hollow your back, and hold. Hips stay on the floor.

Additional Exercises for Riders

Exercise No. 80

Stretching Neck Muscles, Relieving Tension in Neck and Spinal Region

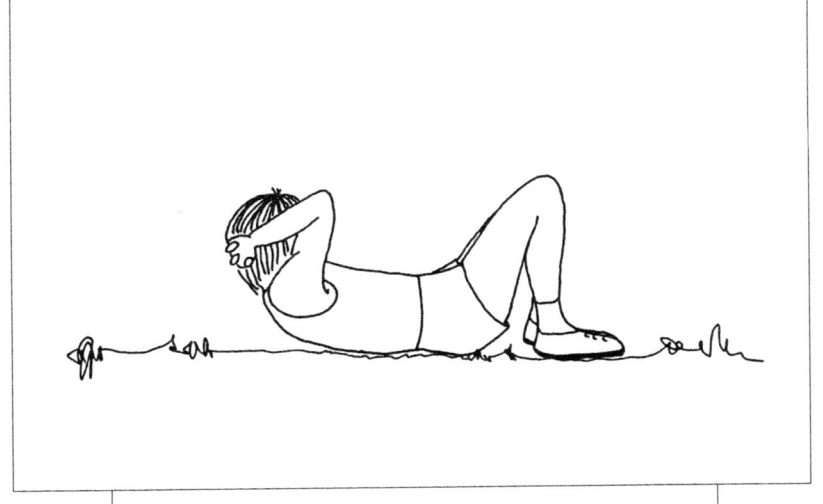

Lie on your back, with feet pulled in almost to your hips. Bring your head forward and hold.

Additional Exercises for Riders

Exercise No. 81

Stretching
Shoulder and Arm Muscles

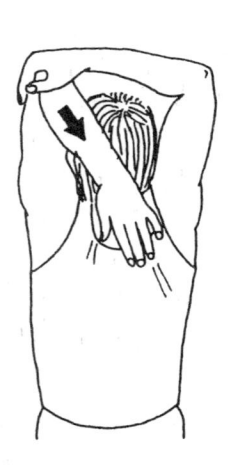

Standing up, push arm behind head in the direction of the shoulder blades. First stretch, then hold. Work on both sides.

Practical Part II

Additional Exercises for Riders

Flexibility and Coordination Exercises

Additional Exercises for Riders

Exercise No. 82

Flexibility of the Pelvis, Improving Coordination

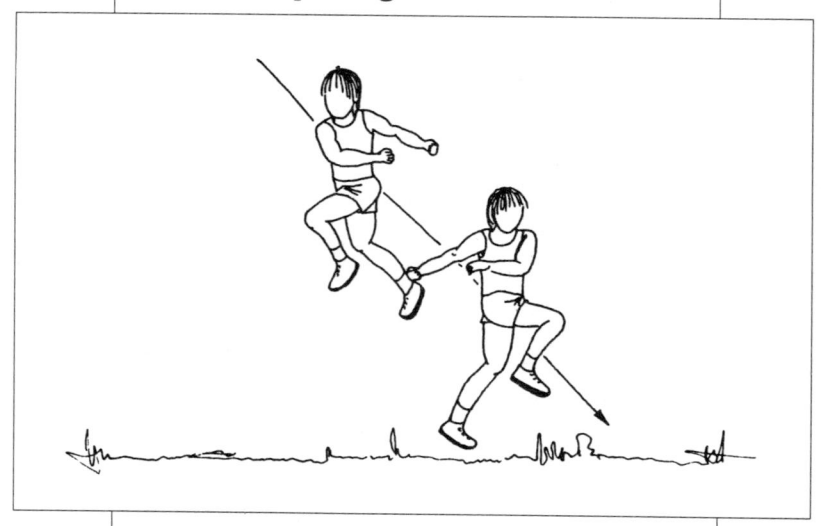

Skip, and alternately pivot in the air to the right, then to the left.

Additional Exercises for Riders

Exercise No. 83

Strengthening the Torso Muscles, Improving Coordination

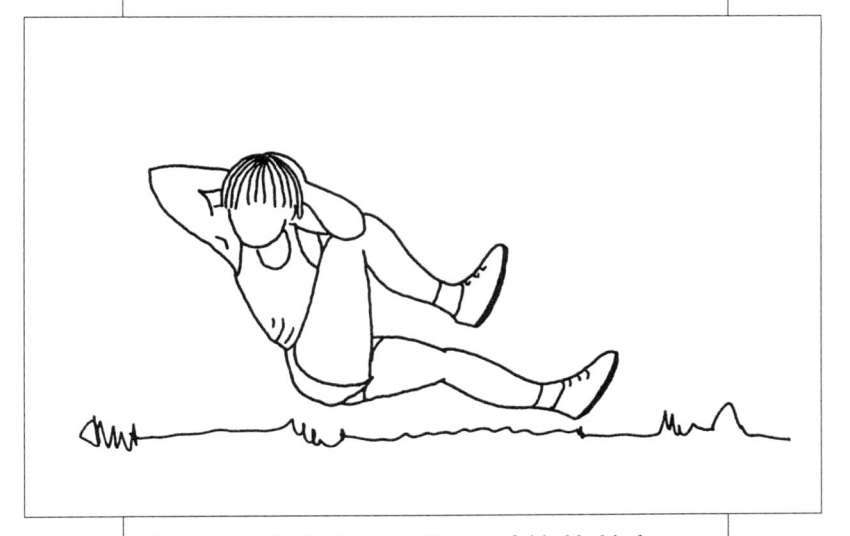

Lie on your back, rise up with arms folded behind your head. While rising, take the left elbow over the right pulled-up knee, alternating right and left.

Additional Exercises for Riders

Exercise No. 84

Flexibility of the Shoulders

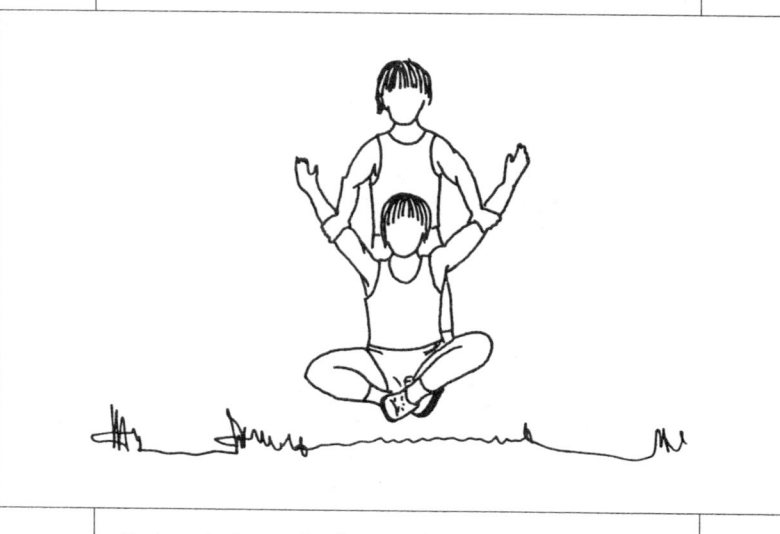

Partner A sits on the floor, and B stands behind her. B's knees are at the shoulder blades of A, with A's arms held up. B gently pulls A's arms backwards, elastically.

Additional Exercises for Riders

Exercise No. 85

Stretching Lower Back Muscles, Relieving Tension in the Loin Region

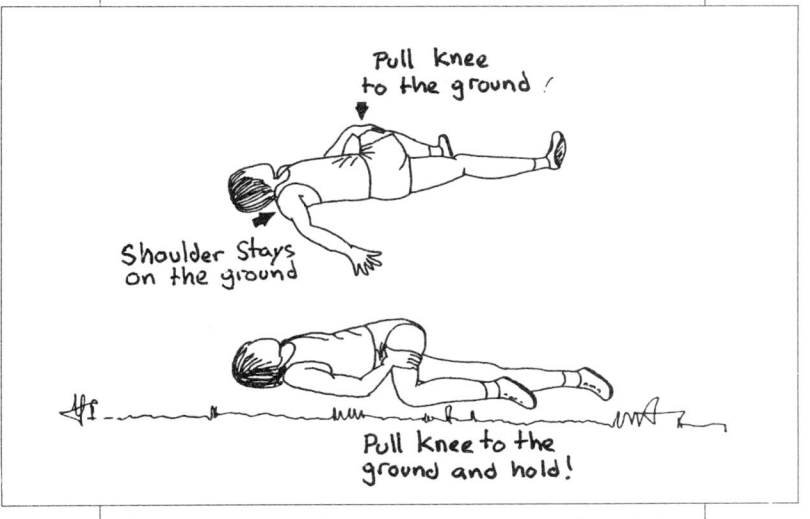

Lie on your back with both shoulders on the floor. Pull your right knee with your left hand to the floor. Repeat on the other side.

Additional Exercises for Riders

Exercise No. 86

Mobility of Pelvic Region, Improving Coordination

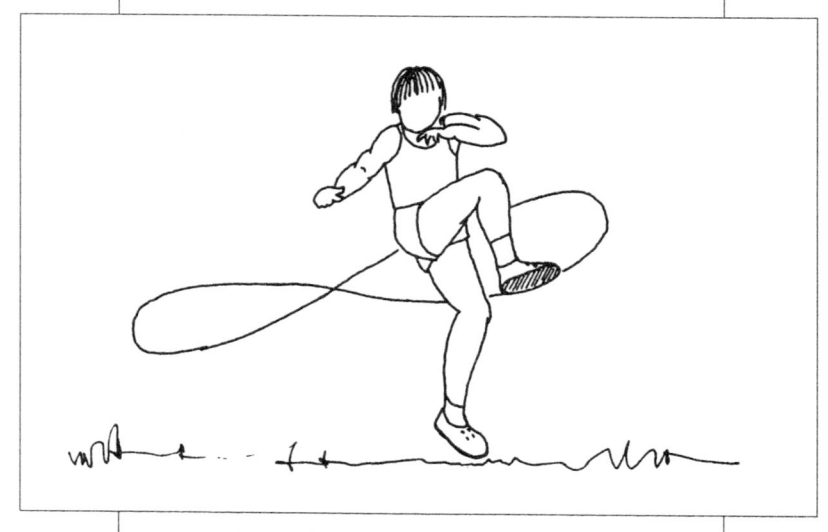

Figure eights: do figure eight circles with each leg several times.

Additional Exercises for Riders

Exercise No. 87

Strengthening the Back Muscles, Improving Mobility of Pelvic Region

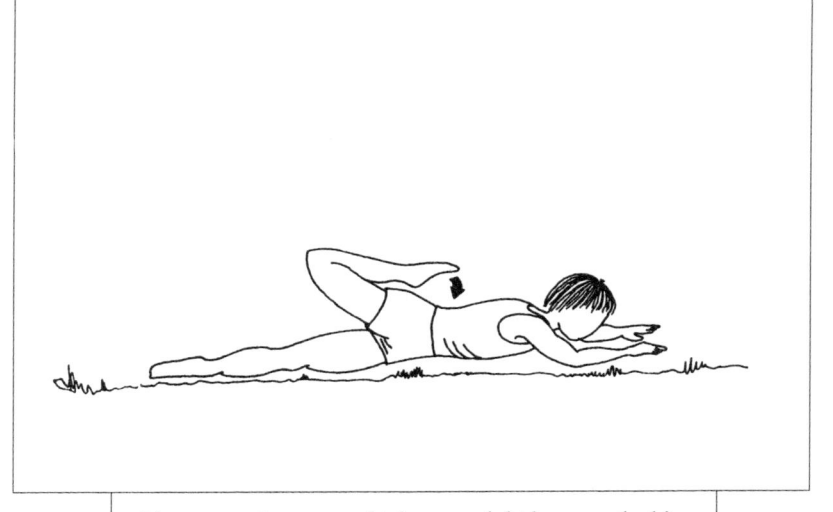

Lie on your tummy, and take your right leg over the hip to the opposite shoulder. Do *not* lift shoulder. Alternate right and left.

Additional Exercises for Riders

Exercise No. 88

Mobility of Pelvic Region

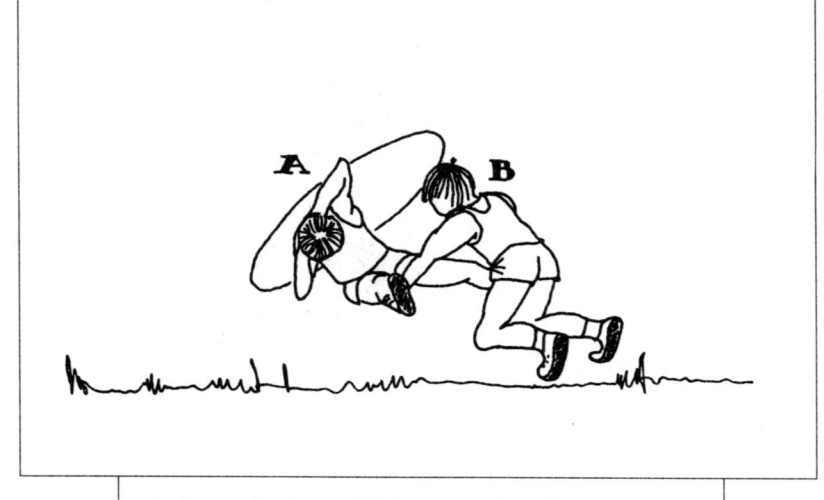

A sits on the floor with legs spread, while B holds A's feet. A moves in circles to both sides.

Additional Exercises for Riders

Exercise No. 89

Mobility of Shoulders

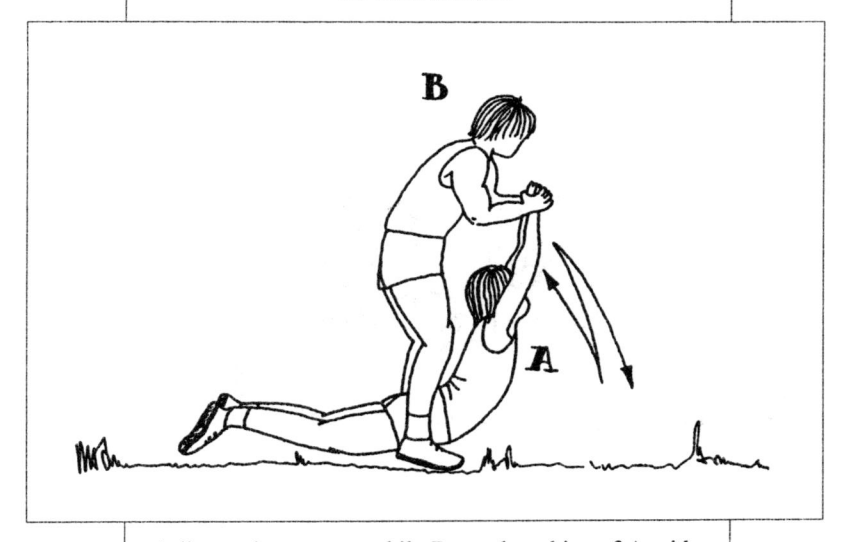

A lies on her tummy while B stands at hips of A with spread legs, rhythmically lifting up A's arms.

Additional Exercises for Riders

Exercise No. 90

Mobility of Spine and Pelvic Region

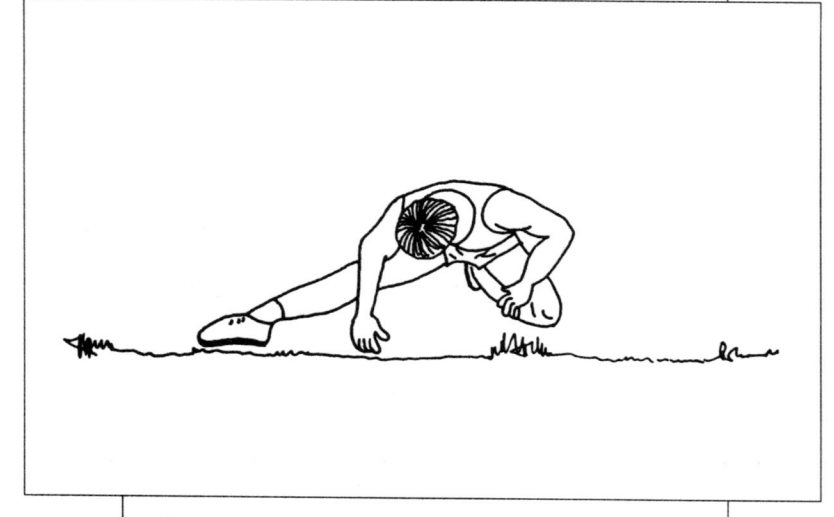

Sit on your heels and bend your body forward. Bend right leg with left leg extended in 90° angle; stretch forward, hold. Alternate

Practical Part III

Additional Exercises for Vaulters

Strengthening Exercises

Additional Exercises for Vaulters

Exercise No. 91

Strengthening the Back

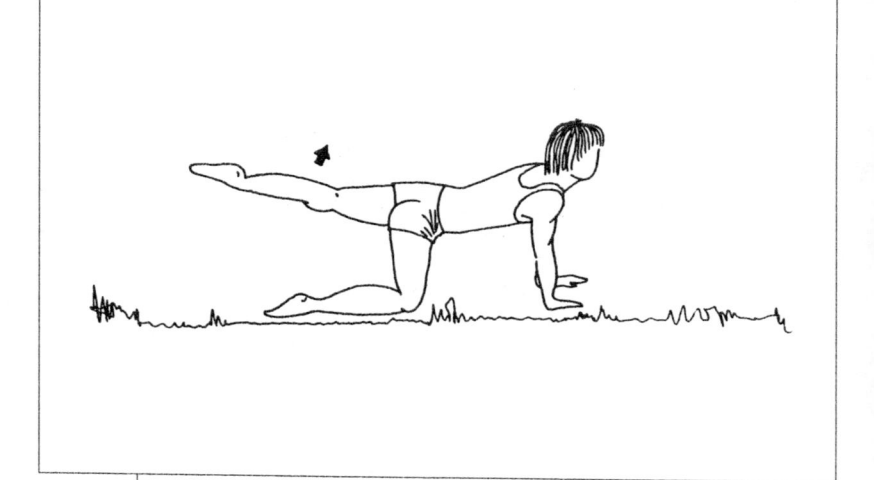

In a one-sided kneestand on the floor, lift and lower one leg, then hold at the highest point. Alternate.

Additional Exercises for Vaulters

Exercise No. 92

Strengthening Stomach Muscles

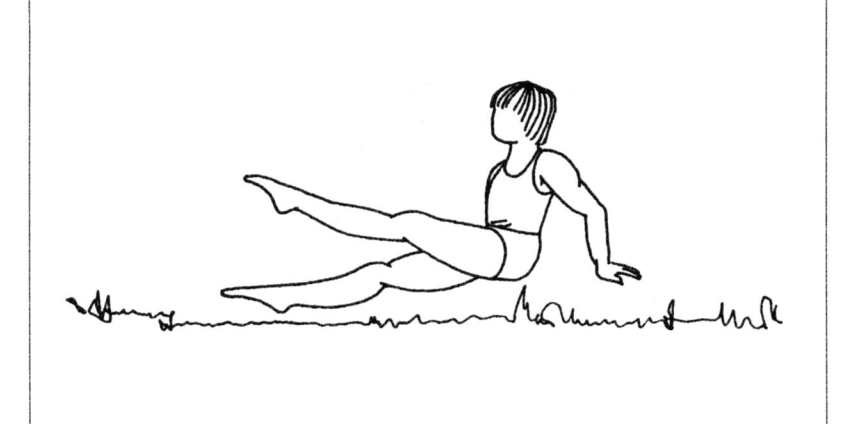

"Windmill" on the floor: while leaning back on both arms with upper body upright, extend your legs. Lift one leg as high as possible; swing to side to an angle of 90°, return to the starting position. Repeat on the other side.

Additional Exercises for Vaulters

Exercise No. 93

Strengthening Stomach and Shoulder Muscles

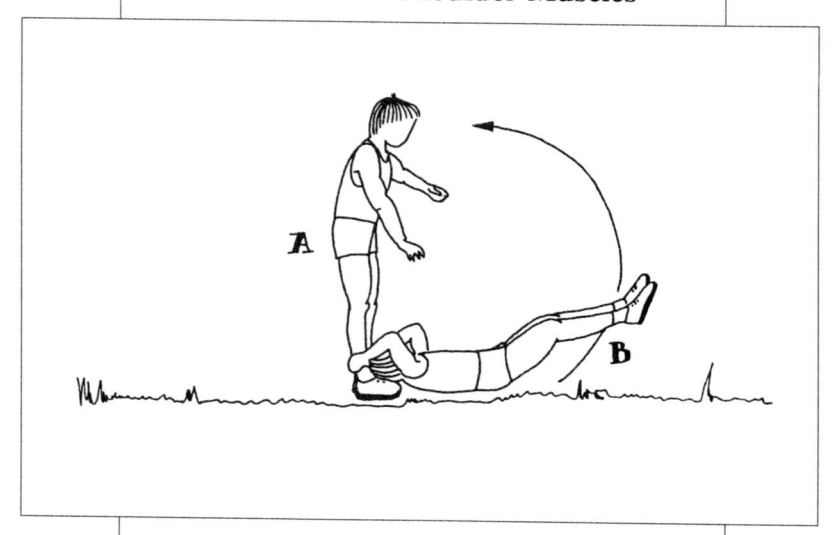

A stands on the floor. B is on her back and holds A's ankles, lifting her legs to a 90° angle. A pushes the legs back and B catches the momentum just before her legs reach the floor.

Additional Exercises for Vaulters

Exercise No. 94

Strengthening Torso Muscles

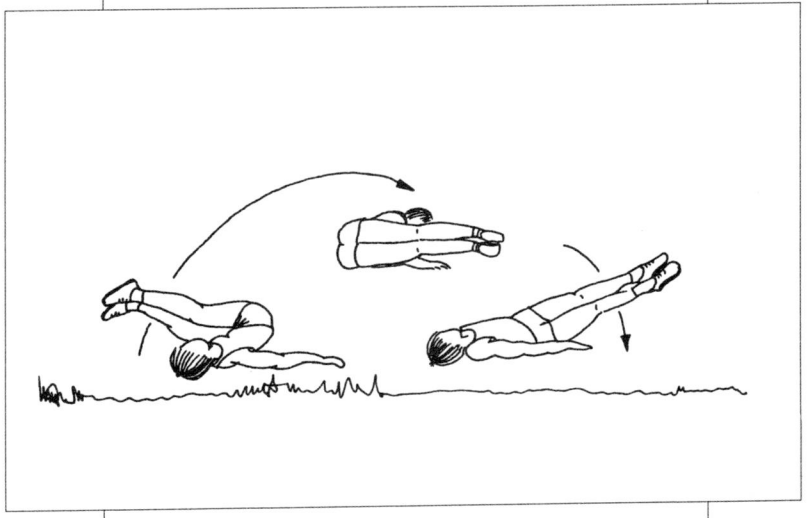

Begin on your back; lift legs closed together over the vertical, from left to right and vice versa.

Additional Exercises for Vaulters

Exercise No. 95

Strengthening Leg Muscles, Balance Training

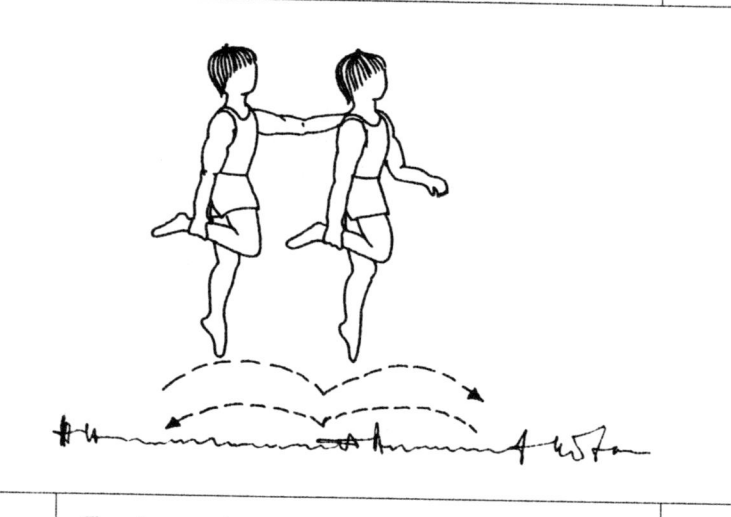

Two (or more) partners stand on one leg and put their hands on the shoulder of the partner in front, while the other hand holds the leg at the ankle. All hop at the same time, forward and backward.

Additional Exercises for Vaulters

Exercise No. 96

Strengthening Arm, Shoulder, and Back Muscles

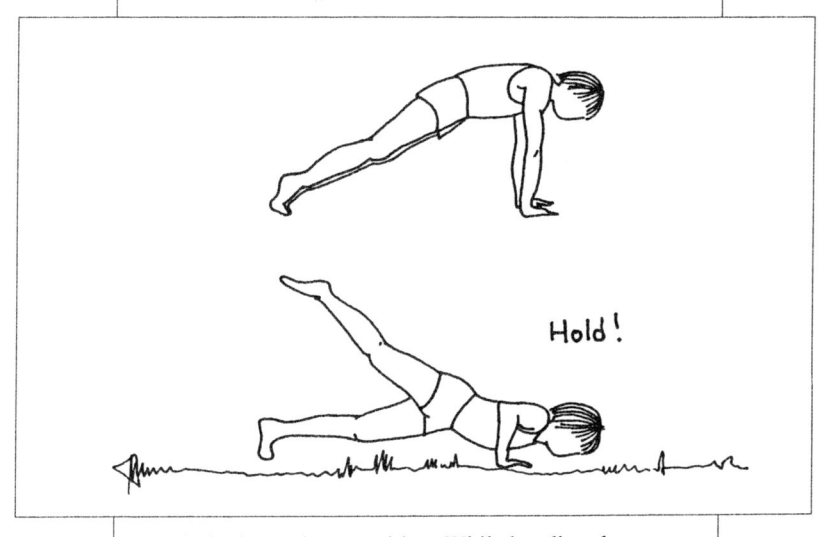

Hold!

Begin in the push-up position. While bending the arms, stretch one leg up and hold. Repeat the excercise, alternating legs.

Additional Exercises for Vaulters

Exercise No. 97

Strengthening Stomach Muscles, Improving Coordination

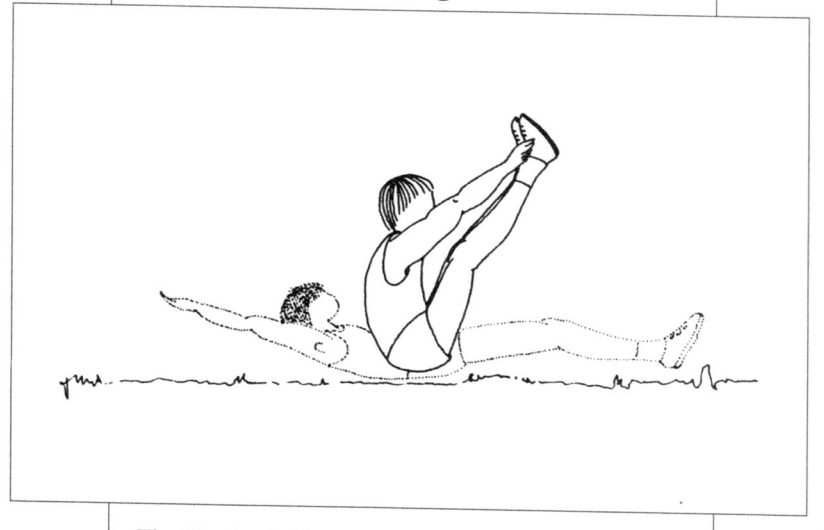

The "Pocket-knife": lift and lower arms and legs at the same time. Always start from a fully stretched position on the floor.

Additional Exercises for Vaulters

Exercise No. 98

Strengthening Arm Muscles and Shoulder Region

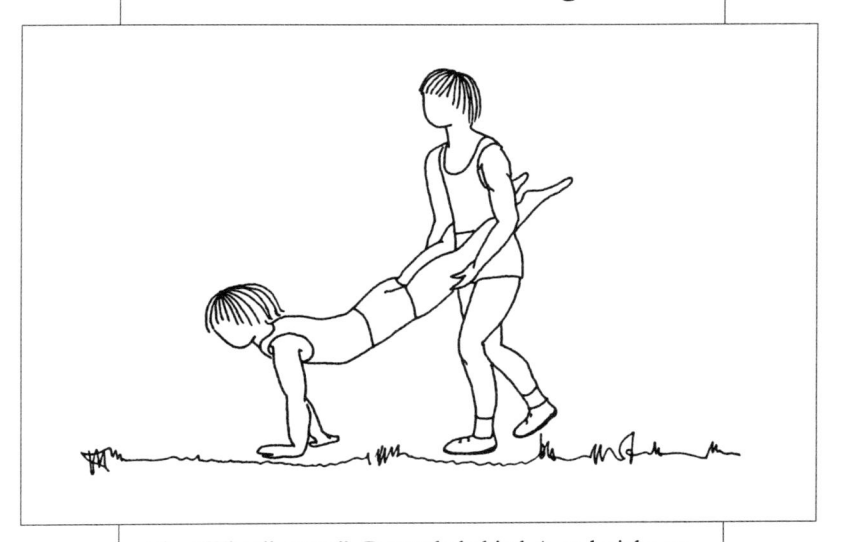

The "Wheelbarrow". B stands behind A and picks up her ankles. A walks forward on her hands. **Note:** Holding the ankles has the best effect, but the seat must always be higher than the shoulders, don't "hang" the back!

Additional Exercises for Vaulters

Exercise No. 99

Strengthening Back Muscles

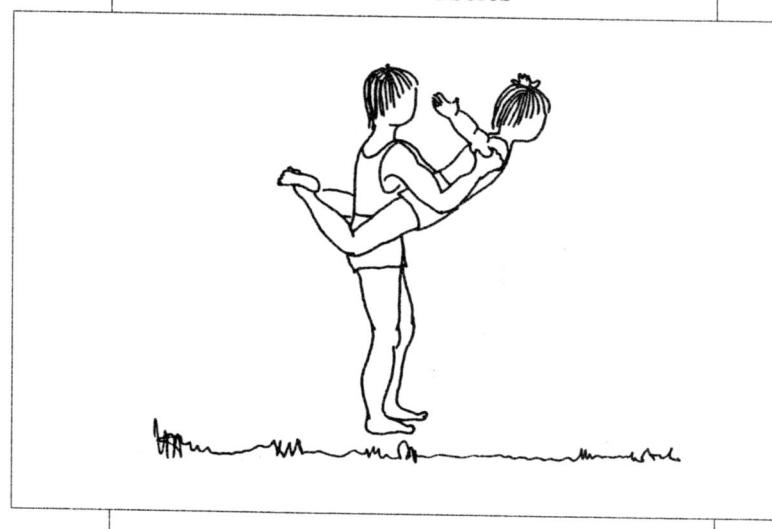

A starts in the push-up position, and B stands behind her. A puts her legs around B's hips, with B holding the upper body of A. A pushes away from the floor as B helps her above the horizontal.

Additional Exercises for Vaulters

Exercise No. 100

Strengthening Arm Muscles, Improving Coordination and Balance

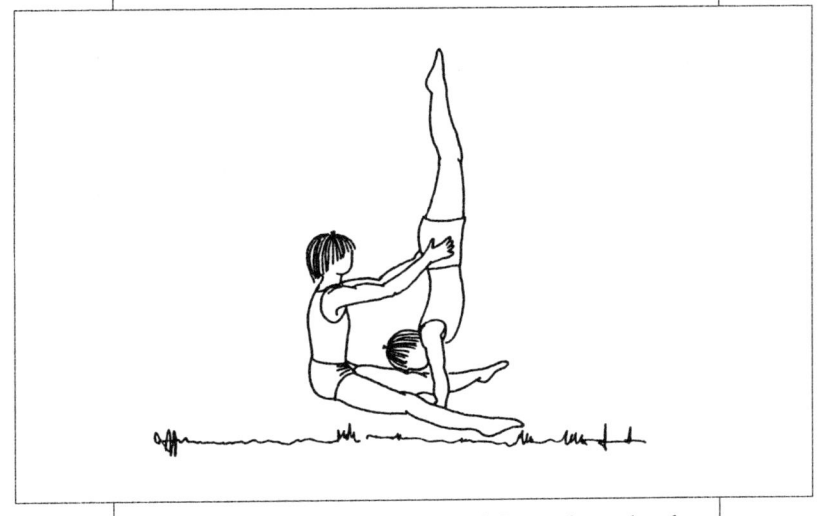

A sits on the floor with legs spread. B gets into a handstand in front of A, and A supports B by her hips. Hold.

Practical Part III

Additional Exercises for Vaulters

Stretching Exercises

Additional Exercises for Vaulters

Exercise No. 101

Stretching Back Muscles and Back Thigh Muscles

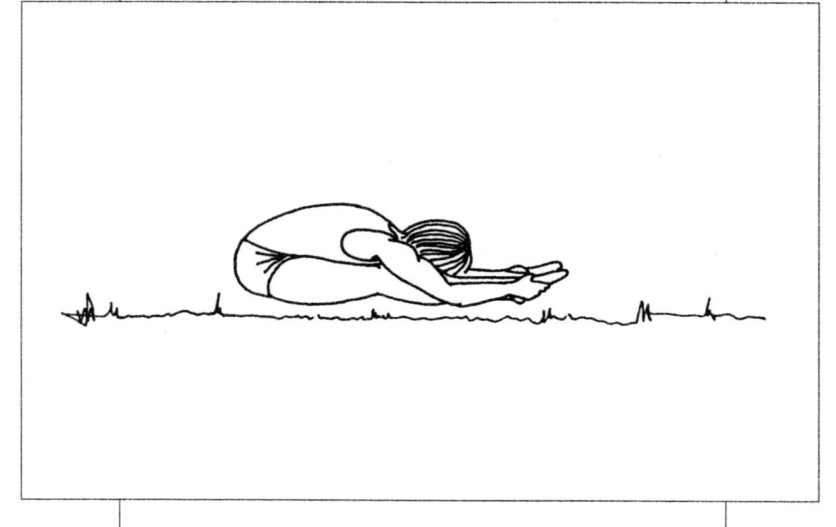

Sit on the floor with legs stretched to the toes. Lower your upper body onto your thighs and hold.

Additional Exercises for Vaulters

Exercise No. 102

Stretching Back Muscles and Back Thigh Muscles

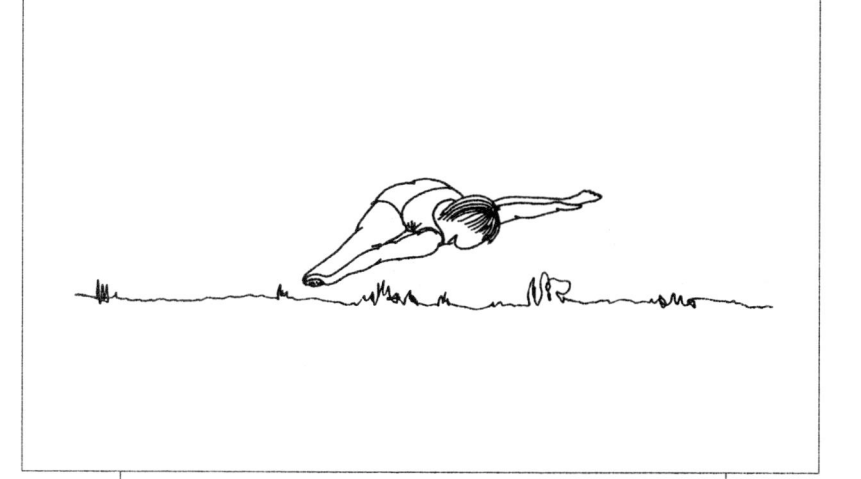

Sit on the floor with legs spread to each side, stretched all the way to the toes. Bend your upper body as far forward as possible; hold.

Additional Exercises for Vaulters

Exercise No. 103

Stretching the Thighs, Mobility of Hip Region

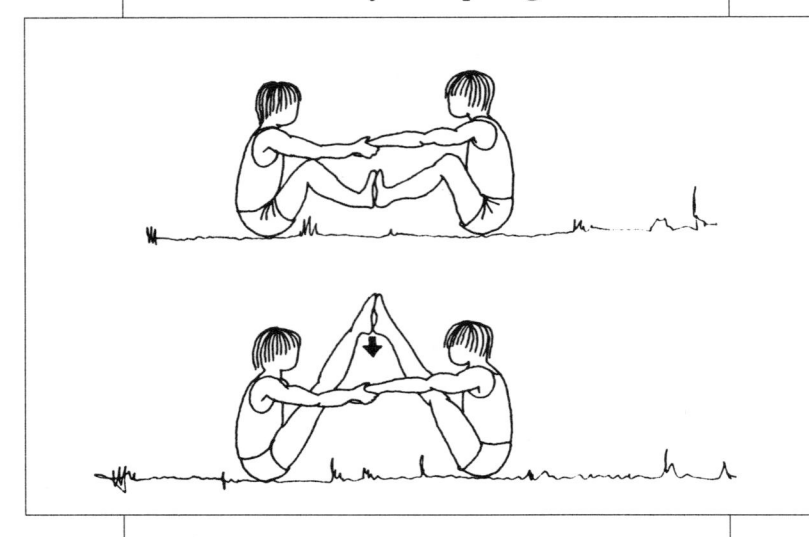

Two partners sit facing each other with legs bent, soles touching, and arms forward while holding hands. Both partners stretch legs up at the same time and lower them again to starting position.

Additional Exercises for Vaulters

Exercise No. 104

Stretching the Leg Muscles
Stretching the Toes

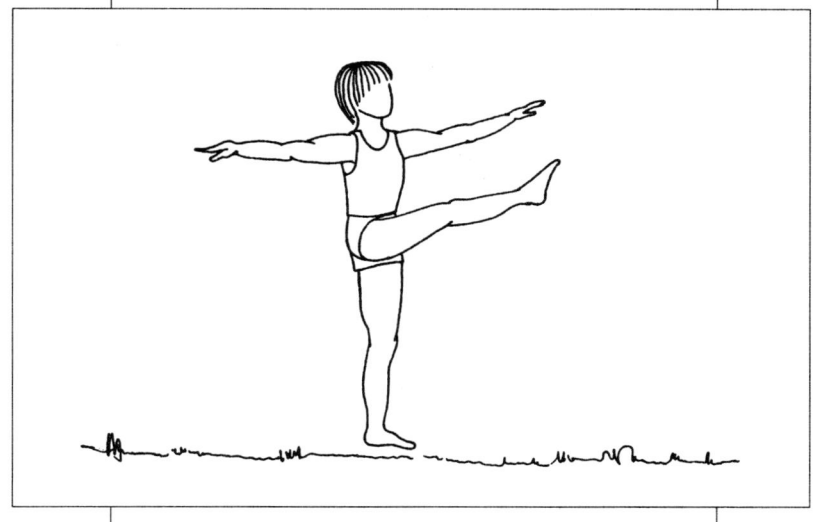

Standing up lift your right stretched leg to your left outstretched arm; alternate both sides.

Additional Exercises for Vaulters

Exercise No. 105

Stretching the Muscles that Bend the Hips

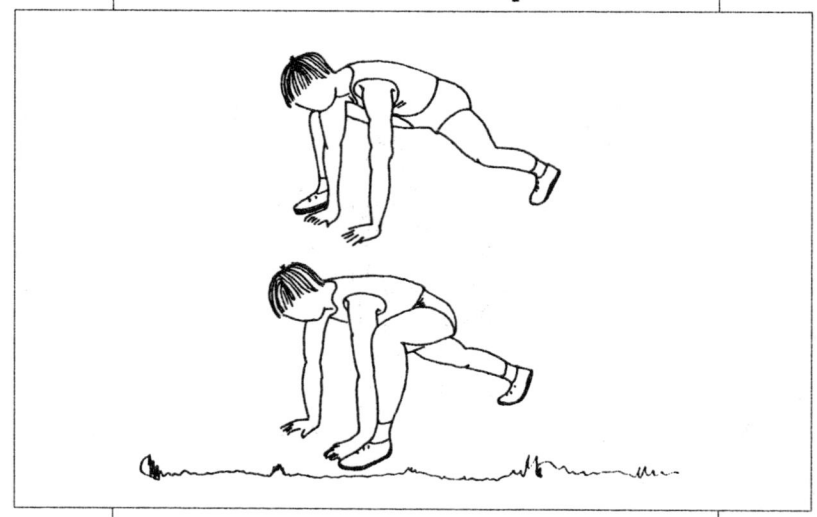

In the push-up position, put your right foot next to your right hand, and hold. Alternate sides.

Additional Exercises for Vaulters

Exercise No. 106

Stretching Shoulder and Leg Muscles

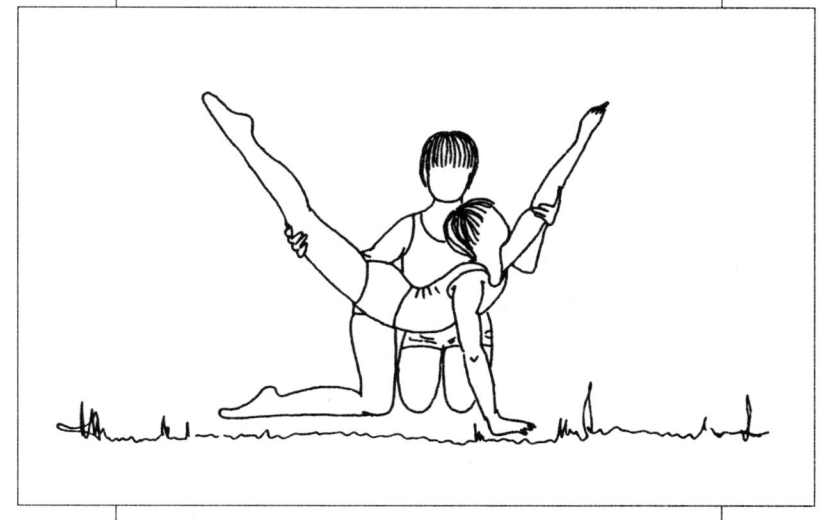

Stretch your arm and leg up with the help of a partner.

Practical Part III

Additional Exercises for Vaulters

Flexibility and Coordination Exercises

Additional Exercises for Vaulters

Exercise No. 107

Coordination (balance), Strengthening Leg Muscles

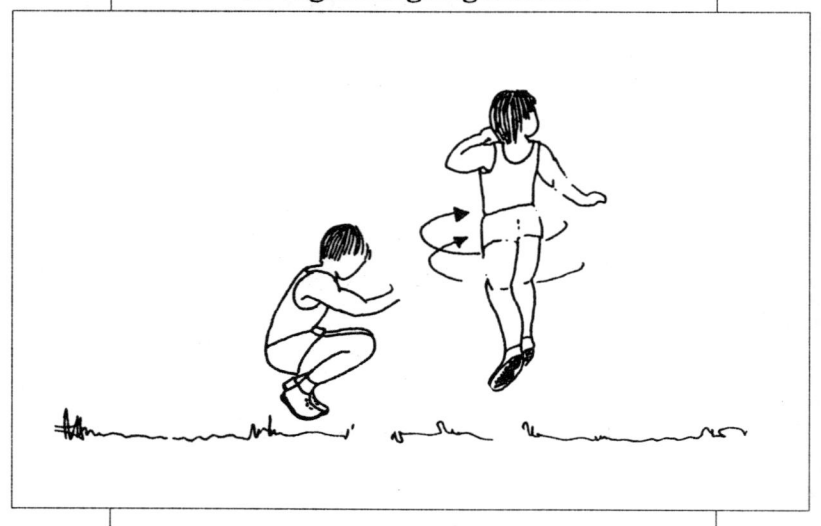

Jump up out of a squatting position while turning right and left.

Additional Exercises for Vaulters

Exercise No. 108

Coordination, Stretching and Strengthening of Torso and Leg Muscles

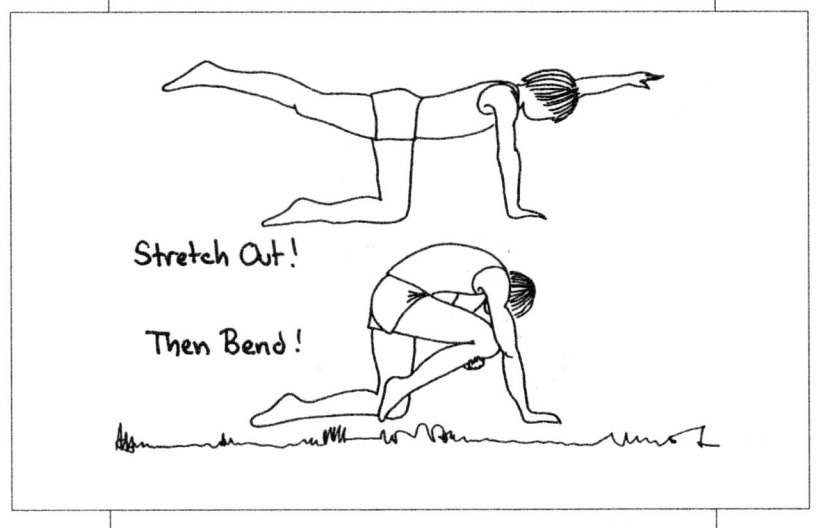

Stretch Out!

Then Bend!

The "Flag": stretch and bend, alternately, hold in the stretched position.

Additional Exercises for Vaulters

Exercise No. 109

Coordination, Strengthening Leg Muscles

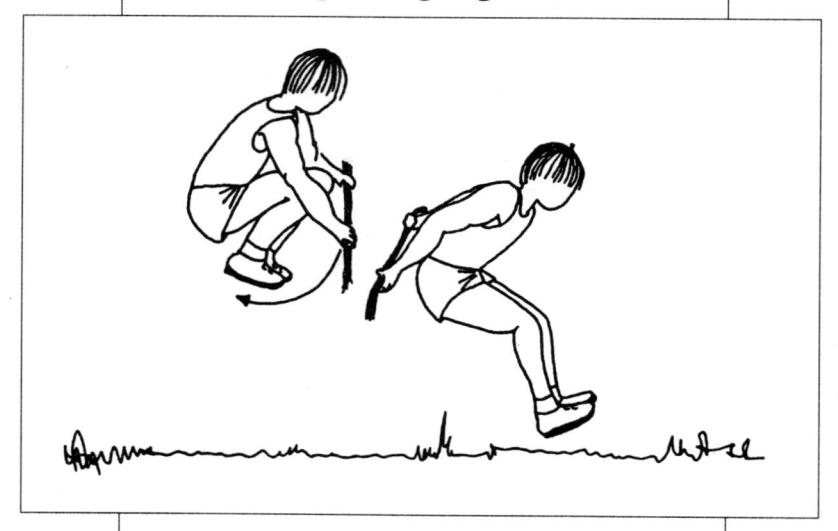

Hold stick or bar shoulder-width, and jump over it with both legs at the same time.

Additional Exercises for Vaulters

Exercise No. 110

Coordination, Strengthening Leg Muscles, Improve Ability to Spread Legs

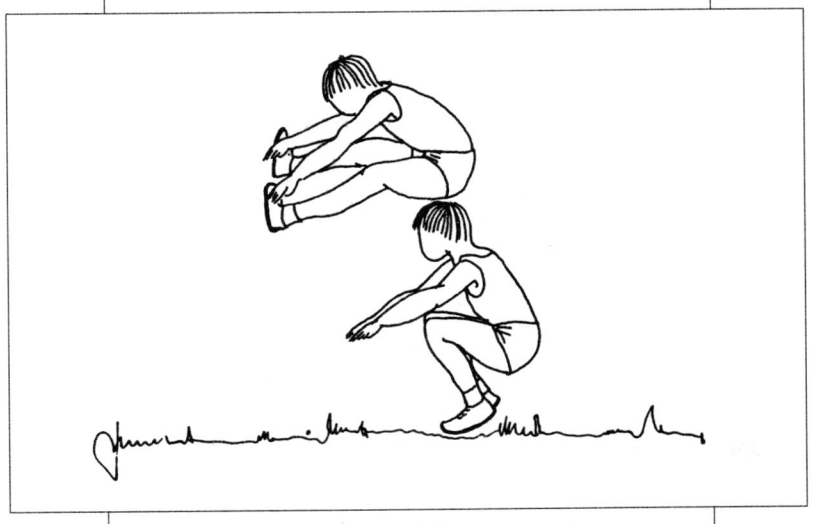

Jump up, lifting both spread legs to spread out arms, keeping upper body upright.

Additional Exercises for Vaulters

Exercise No. 111

Balance

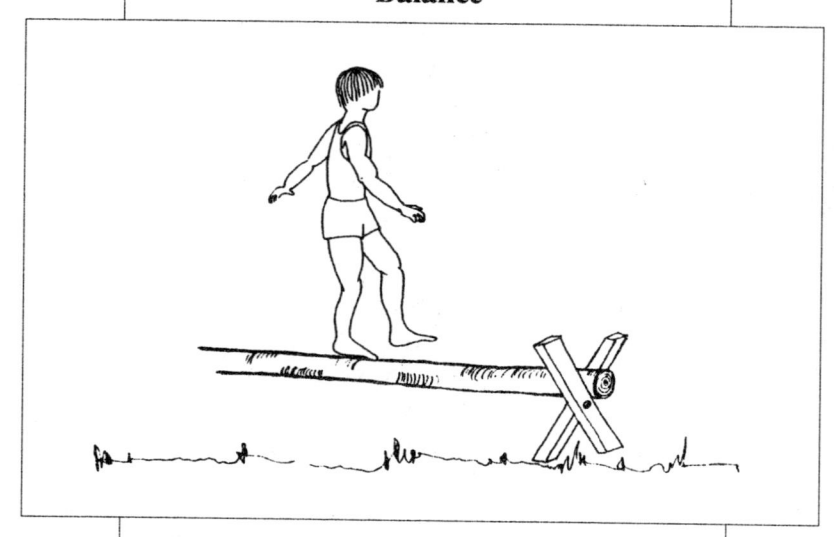

Balance on a cavaletti. Have a partner try to disturb your balance while you recover.

Additional Exercises for Vaulters

Exercise No. 112

Balance

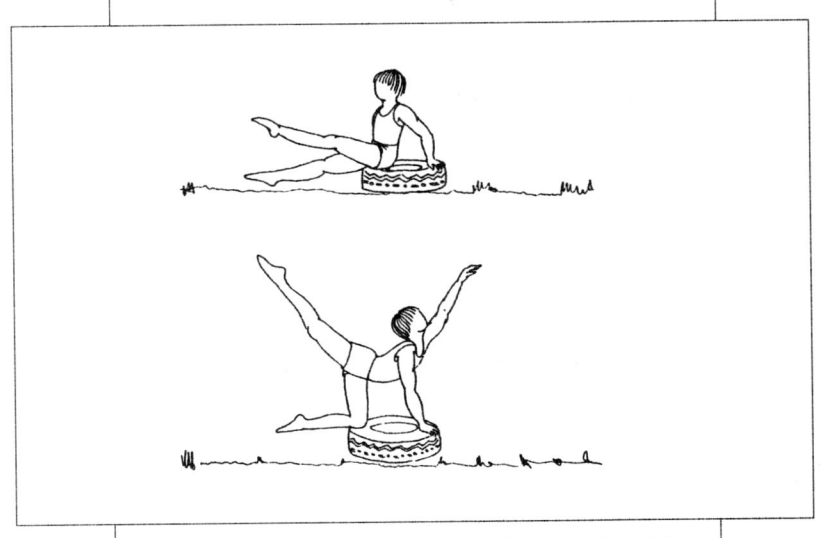

A tries to balance ("flag" or "windmill") on a tire while B moves the tire trying to unbalance A.

Additional Exercises for Vaulters

Exercise No. 113

Balance, Strengthening Leg Muscles

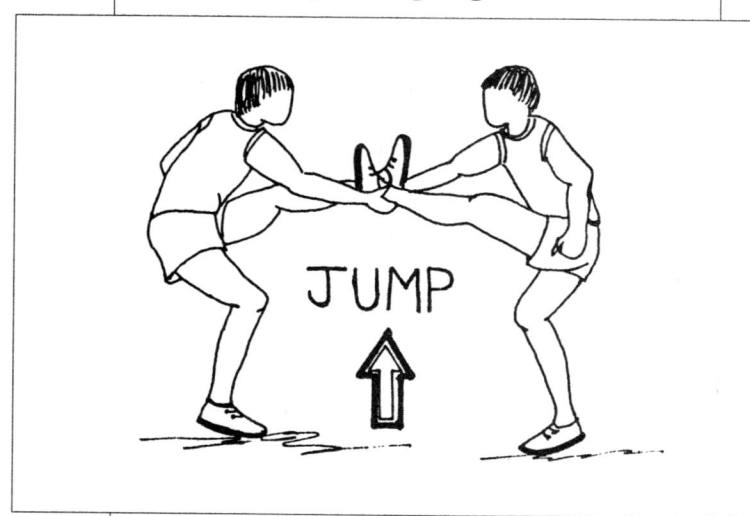

One-legged junping: A's right hand holds B's left leg and vice versa; they try to jump high with toes stretched.

Additional Exercises for Vaulters

Exercise No. 114

Mobility of Ankles

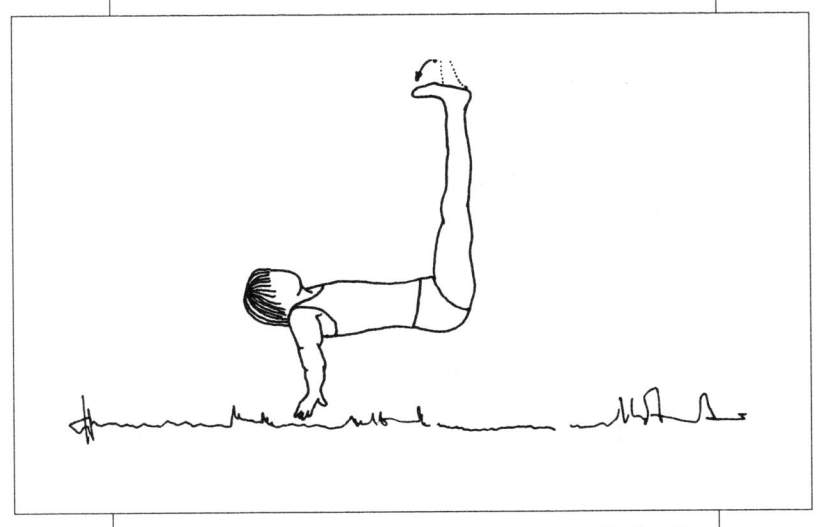

Lying on your back, with legs up in a 90° angle, bend and stretch your feet.

Additional Exercises for Vaulters

Exercise No. 115

Mobility of Ankles

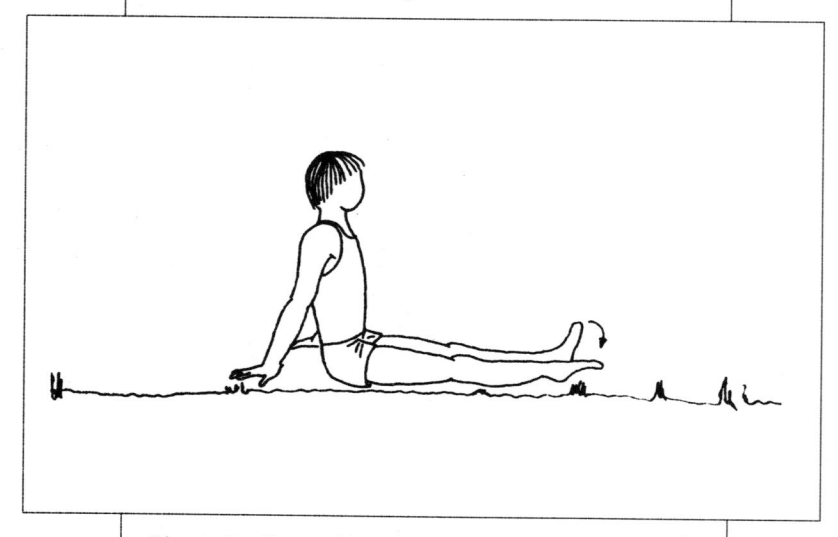

Sit on the floor with legs stretched. Stretch right foot and bend left foot at the same time, and vice versa.

Additional Exercises for Vaulters

Exercise No. 116

Mobility of Ankles

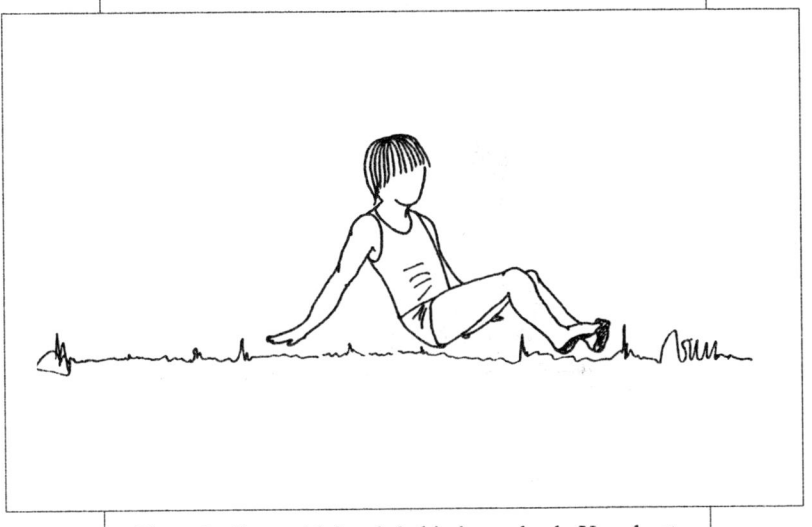

Sit on the floor with hands behind your back. Your bent legs do not touch the floor. Circle feet inwards and outwards.

Additional Exercises for Vaulters

Exercise No. 117

Flexibility of Hips, Stretching Back Thigh Muscles

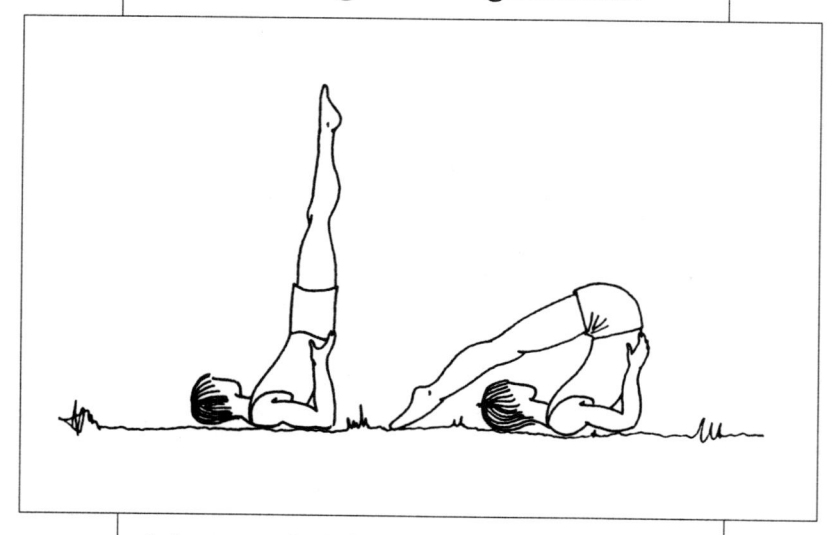

Lying on your back, lift up legs to the "candle" position. Bring your stretched legs behind your head onto the floor and hold.

Additional Exercises for Vaulters

Exercise No. 118

Flexibility of the Hips, Stretching Back Thigh Muscles

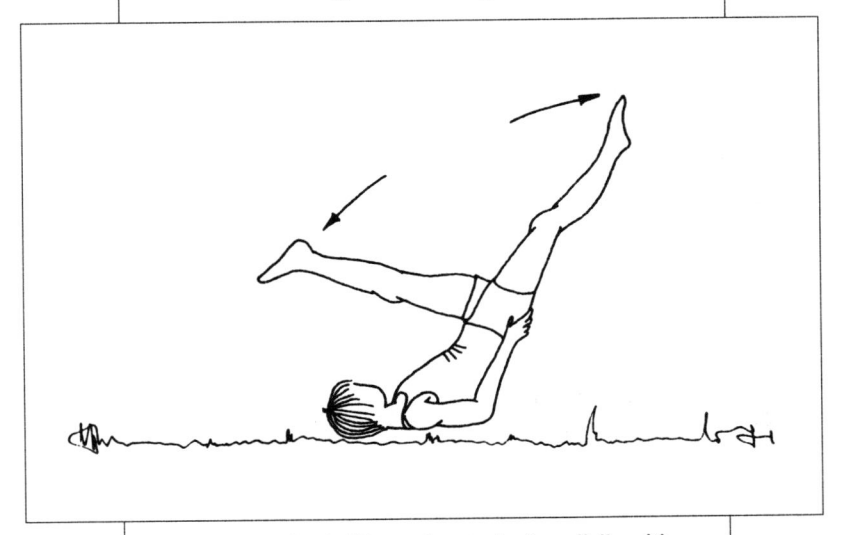

Lying on your back, lift your legs to the "candle" position. Put your right, then left leg behind your head on the floor, and hold.

Additional Exercises for Vaulters

Exercise No. 119

Flexibility of the Spine

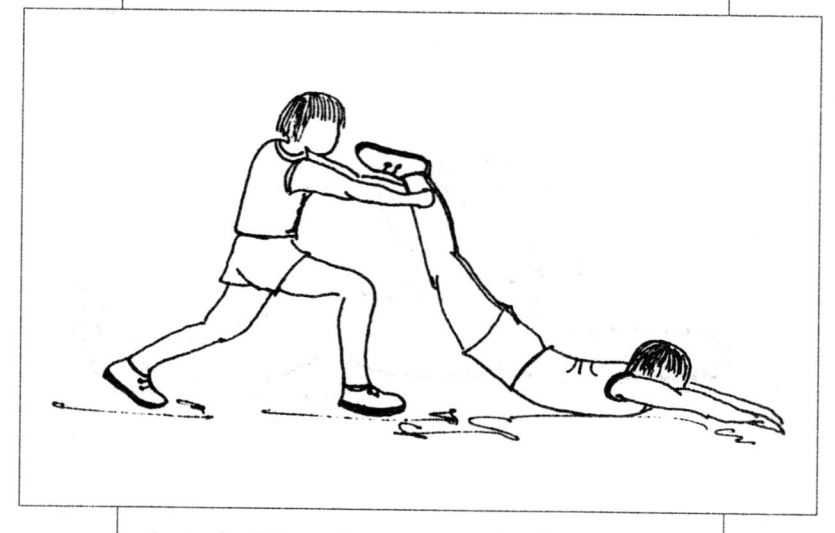

A stands, B is on her tummy on the floor. A pushes against B's stretched legs, and moves them up and down, at first gently, then more vigorously.

Additional Exercises for Vaulters

Exercise No. 120

Flexibility of the Pelvis, Stretching Back and Leg Muscles

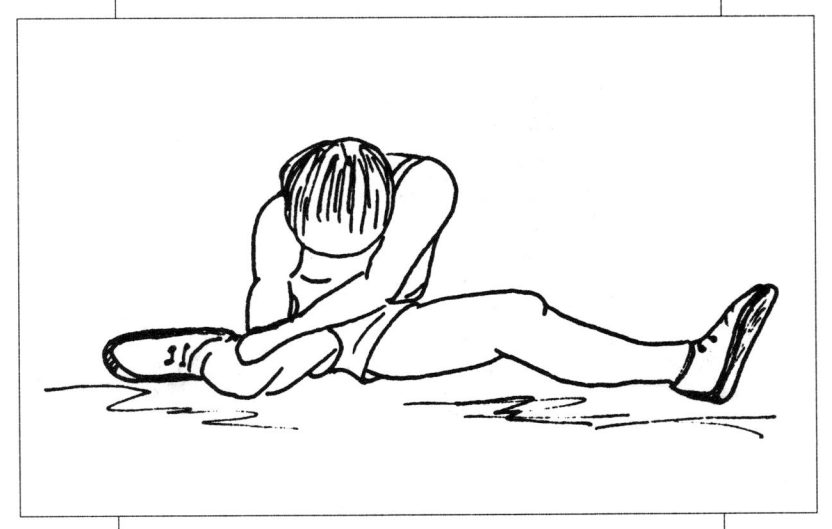

From the hurdle seat position with one leg stretched forward, bend your upper body to the floor, seesaw and hold.